Integrative Health Nursing Interventions for Vulnerable Populations

Amber Vermeesch

Editor

Integrative Health Nursing Interventions for Vulnerable Populations

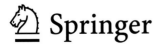 Springer

Editor
Amber Vermeesch
School of Nursing
University of Portland
Portland, OR
USA

ISBN 978-3-030-60042-6   ISBN 978-3-030-60043-3   (eBook)
https://doi.org/10.1007/978-3-030-60043-3

This Springer imprint is published by the registered company Springer Nature Switzerland AG
The registered company address is: Gewerbestrasse 11, 6330 Cham, Switzerland

Foreword

The US healthcare system has long struggled with providing care that is affordable, accessible, and delivered in a manner that is responsive to the needs of its most vulnerable populations. Today, as we face what seems to be a perfect storm where a pandemic challenges the very foundation of our social fabric and our collective biomedical knowledge and reveals the devastating effects of systemic racism and a legacy of environmental neglect and exploitation on health and well-being, these authors offer unique perspectives and strategies based on nursing's perennial wisdom that embraces an integrative approach to care.

Integrative nursing calls us to care for the whole person, recognizing that context, including the social, relational, geopolitical, cultural, and temporal aspects of a person's life, frames both the interventions that we choose and the manner in which we counsel and guide individuals, families, and communities. Further, an integrative approach embraces the complexities of our times, encouraging nurses to identify ways to deliver care in a more just and culturally safe manner and to recognize and address the effects that chronic unremitting stress has on the health and well-being of all patients. While there is increasingly irrefutable evidence that chronic stress is the underlying mechanism for most of our most devastating chronic illnesses, there is growing consensus that vulnerable populations face an unequal burden of chronic stress given the challenges of their everyday life. This book addresses those challenges and provides guidelines for nurses and other healthcare professionals seeking to improve the effectiveness of their interventions.

Embracing integrative nursing's belief that people have an innate healing capacity that requires a provider that is supportive and generative rather than directive and prescriptive, the authors provide guidelines to reduce stress and build body-mind-spirit resilience in different populations. Likewise, their approach to symptom management aligns with the integrative belief that interventions should be individually tailored and employ the least intensive therapeutic strategy so as to minimize additional insult and injury.

This is a very welcome addition to the growing integrative healthcare literature and a much-needed examination of nursing's role in the integrative care of vulnerable populations. My hope is that the information found within these chapters stimulates ongoing dialogue about the care we must provide to those entrusted to us and serious reflection about what actions the profession of nursing must take in order to ensure that all persons have the resources needed to achieve optimal health and well-being. As this book so eloquently demonstrates, integrative nursing addresses accessibility, quality, safety, patient-centeredness, and affordability—all qualities that our healthcare system desperately needs in these historic and unprecedented times.

Mary Koithan
College of Nursing
Washington State University
Pullman, WA, USA

Preface

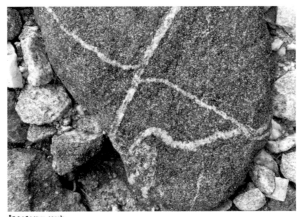

°2019 Vermeesch

There are many winding paths to health –
be a pathfinder

The final preparation of this book, during the summer of 2020, coincides with multiple events in our world, the effects of which have yet to be fully determined. The intersection of the COVID-19 pandemic, the escalating fight against racial inequities, global warming and the effects of the environment on health, and the struggle for accessible healthcare to optimize wellness will shape our world in ways we cannot yet predict.

This book provides a timely opportunity for dissemination of what my colleagues across the United States have been working tirelessly on this past year, and in some cases, much longer. This is a collection of work designed to provide guidance for implementing integrative health nursing interventions for educators, practitioners, clinicians, researchers, and students to better serve vulnerable populations in multiple contexts. This book is of interest to nursing educators, practitioners, and students. Researchers and scholars will find this an appealing and refreshing approach in diminishing health inequities among vulnerable populations. This book informs clinicians, faculty, practitioners, and students working with vulnerable and underserved populations on effective wellness strategies to address inadequate nutrition, physical activity promotion, and perceived stress reduction through an integrative health nursing framework. Beginning with an overview of cultural humility, health inequities, and social justice to justify the use of an integrative health nursing framework, the book continues by addressing interventions to reduce perceived stress, promote nutrition strategies, and physical activity interventions.

As nurses, integrative health is in the very marrow of our bones. From the time of Florence Nightingale, nurses have been unifying heretofore separate aspects of health in their service to the vulnerable in an integrative approach. This work is ongoing as we work within existing healthcare systems. In the United States, Dr. Andrew Weil is widely recognized as the father of integrative health and has accomplished much to advance mainstream awareness and acceptance of integrative health. The National Institutes of Health and the University of Arizona Andrew Weil Center for Integrative Medicine maintain that integrative health and medicine emphasizes the mental, emotional, functional, spiritual, social, and community aspects of the healing process in which patients and practitioners are partners. This book embodies this viewpoint.

I would like to extend immense gratitude to Springer publisher for the opportunity to bring you this book, to my collaborating authors for their words of wisdom, patience, and flexibility while creating this work during the COVID-19 pandemic, and to my beautiful family, my rocks, Jarod, and Sora, for their unflagging support and patience during the development of this book.

Portland, OR, USA   Amber Vermeesch

Contents

Cultural Humility

1

Isabelle Soulé

1.1 Introduction

In the twenty-first century, health has become a shared global responsibility, involving the need for equitable access to essential care for all individuals. Statements by leading professional organizations clearly entitle all people of the world equally to civil, economic, social, and cultural rights, including the right to health (ANA 2018; ICN 2018; WHO 2018). Indeed, all human rights are best thought of as inseparable because poor health has harmful effects on other basic human rights such as safety, education, dignity, and meaningful participation in society.

Working effectively with vulnerable populations is complex and requires moving beyond a biomedical view of health to understand the larger contextual factors that influence health and well-being. This paradigm shift is fueled by (a) the rapidly shifting demographics of the USA to a more ethnically, racially, and linguistically diverse population; (b) recognition of the important role culture plays in healthcare provision and reception; (c) an increased evidence base substantiating long-standing health and healthcare disparities; and (d) ethical and legal mandates from professional organizations and accrediting bodies requiring professional competencies for healthcare education, professional practice, and healthcare organizations (Chang et al. 2012; Fisher-Borne et al. 2015). It is now recognized that a continuation of a singular way of thinking or acting based on a singular set of cultural norms is not only unethical, it is also unprofitable. Unethical, because it does not provide accommodation for unique beliefs, values, or traditions. Unprofitable, because clients and communities seek out alternatives to healthcare providers and systems who do not listen carefully, are not aligned with their wishes, and discriminate against them.

Ethnic, spiritual, sexual, gender, and other dimensions of difference are *not* problems; however, prejudice, discrimination, conflict, and health disparities *are*

I. Soulé (✉)
School of Nursing, University of Portland, Portland, OR, USA
e-mail: soule@up.edu

© Springer Nature Switzerland AG 2021
A. Vermeesch (ed.), *Integrative Health Nursing Interventions for Vulnerable Populations*, https://doi.org/10.1007/978-3-030-60043-3_1

problems. *Health disparities,* defined as the differences in the incidence, prevalence, mortality, and burden of diseases, are a particular type of health difference related to the conditions in which a person makes choices and are closely linked with social, economic, educational, or environmental disadvantage. Collectively, these influences are referred to as *social determinants of health* and generate a context in which individuals and communities experience health and illness including the dynamic interplay among ethnicity, gender, socioeconomic status, and social rank. It also includes the degree of choice they have regarding access to healthcare providers and systems who understand and value them (de Chesnay and Anderson 2016; IOM 2003). Additionally, *healthcare disparities*, the discriminatory and/or preferential treatment of clients and communities by healthcare providers play an important part in continuing to privilege some groups, often at the expense of others (Masters et al. 2019).

Privilege, a result of being part of a mainstream or valued group, can include aspects such as age, appearance, ethnicity, gender, nationality, physical ability, socioeconomic status, educational level, sexual orientation, professional status, and spiritual practice among others. Consequently, diverse and therefore vulnerable, in the context of dominant US culture, is generally thought of as non-white, non-Western, non-heterosexual, non-English-speaking, and non-Christian. Evidence clearly demonstrates that groups who experience discrimination have direct and devastating effects on their physical and mental health as well as lower overall quality of life that includes social stigma, higher rates of ill-health, and higher rates of risk behaviors including self-harm (de Chesnay and Anderson 2016). When underlying biases are not conscientiously examined for the impact that they have on the delivery of care, healthcare providers may inadvertently contribute to disparities by playing a dual role in attempting to reduce health disparities at the same time they are unwittingly maintaining them (Fisher-Borne et al. 2015). Health professionals are now being called upon to understand the larger context in which vulnerable communities live and make choices and to begin thinking differently and "being" differently as they partner with them toward optimal health, as they define it.

1.2   Cultural Competence to Cultural Humility

Over the past 30 years, an extensive body of literature on cultural competence has been generated to support the need for understanding, planning, implementing, evaluating, and refining cultural care. Although there are many definitions, *cultural competence* is generally thought of as the knowledge, skills, and attitudes that enable a health professional or system to provide meaningful, supportive, and beneficial healthcare that preserves a client and community's human rights and dignity (AAN 1992). Traditionally, cultural competence trainings and professional books on caring for the *cultural* client relied primarily on a description of the needs, behaviors, and cultural values of ethnic minorities in order to educate health professionals about the health beliefs and practices of diverse groups. Admittedly, over time this work has been fruitful, resulting in improved resources of many kinds including educational trainings, interpreter services, informative websites, and a greater awareness of the impact of culture on health and illness. However, unexamined assumptions underpinning the concept of cultural competence including a narrow and limiting view of what constitutes culture, reinforce stereotypes rather than engendering respect as originally intended (Gregg and Saha 2006).

Furthermore, the recurrent appeal to health professionals to be sensitive to the cultural context, beliefs, values, and behaviors of clients and communities implicitly denotes culture as a feature residing outside of the healthcare professional and healthcare system. Consequently, when the focus of cultural knowledge is outward, toward the client, the implied corollary belief is that biomedicine, healthcare education, and the US culture in general, where most of the cultural competence literature has emerged, are culture-neutral. This blind spot that fails to also identify the beliefs, behaviors, and customs in the culture of biomedicine, health professional education, and the USA is a major flaw in the cultural competence literature, as each of these cultures merits careful examination as they are not neutral backgrounds against which other cultures can be measured (Gray and Thomas 2005; Hassouneh 2008). Importantly, an outward focus on the beliefs, customs, and traditions of immigrant, refugee, or ethnic minority groups can obscure the interlocking systems and oppressive relations that establish and maintain systems of imbalanced power in which certain groups are systematically privileged and certain groups are systematically devalued (Drevdahl et al. 2008).

Cultural humility is a distinctive paradigm that moves beyond cultural competence to core tenets including (a) lifelong commitment to self-reflection and self-critique, (b) leveling the power differential present between healthcare provider/healthcare organization and client/community, and (c) building mutually beneficial, high-quality partnerships (Dunn and Soulé 2016; Tervalon and Murray-Garcia 1998). Cultural humility is based on passive volition, receptivity, and a willingness to learn from the lived experience of others. Cultural humility requires open-mindedness and open-heartedness and asks questions rather than gives answers. Providers who practice cultural humility demonstrate intellectual, attitudinal, and behavioral flexibility and are able to interact in a non-judgmental way with individuals who have widely different values, beliefs, and worldviews than their own. They are skillful at challenging their own beliefs to move toward more respectful, inclusive healthcare practices, honoring the vulnerable individual or community as experts in their own experience.

Topics such as humility, not often discussed in professional circles, are not simply overlooked but may be perceived in opposition to competence, professionalism, and professional practice as they exist in the US healthcare system today. This division inevitably creates a gap between the values of healthcare professionals and the values of the community within which a professional works. Healthcare providers are most often educated to think of themselves as "expert knowers" without concomitantly acknowledging the inherent wisdom in the lived experience of clients and communities, and, in particular, vulnerable groups. Because many health professionals are educated to think in these terms, they may be quick to misunderstand or reject teachings that offer an unrecognized set of values or alternate set of truths.

Moreover, building partnerships where health professionals respect the expertise of the client and community in their own healthcare decisions runs contrary to how professionalism is taught and role modeled in our schools and professions today (Abdul-Raheem 2018; Benner et al. 2009; Betancourt and Maina 2004).

Cultural arrogance can be thought of as exaggerating our own importance, diminishing the values and beliefs of others, norming of values and beliefs that mirror our own or mainstream communities, and misusing our power and privilege, perhaps unwittingly, in ways that harm vulnerable clients and communities. Arrogance limits our ability to perceive alternatives, diminishes the value in diverse perspectives, and blocks the pathway toward high-quality relationships making it difficult if not impossible to negotiate a collaborative plan of care. Becoming equal partners with our clients and communities is not a natural outcome of most healthcare education, and will require a transformational shift in the way health education and health systems function to bring about this profound and necessary evolution.

1.3   Self-Reflection and Self-Critique

Developing self-awareness is the first step toward disrupting systems of oppression that generate unjust and harmful health disparities and healthcare disparities. Awareness is best understood as simultaneous discernment of self and others and can be represented on a continuum ranging from a lack of awareness (mindlessness, reactivity, impediment of a specific mindset and entrenchment or one-sidedness) on one end to self-awareness (mindful, receptive to the lived experience of others, flexibility, and an ability to imagine from multiple perspectives) on the other. When we lack self-awareness, and are out of touch with our own experiences, we are unable to learn from them, and will find it difficult if not impossible to attune to the experiences of others (Seigel 2010). Conscious awareness enables us to identify ingrained behaviors, be more intentionally aware of how we interact with others and become more sensitive to the unique lived worlds of those around us. Because we do not know what we do not know, a lifelong commitment to self-reflection and self-critique requires a proactive stance including the willingness and courage to uncover unconscious bias and prejudice that influence our ability to work effectively with vulnerable clients and communities. It also allows us to recognize how systems of oppression work and our particular roles in maintaining them. The purpose of self-reflection and self-critique is to identify how we think and act to change the way we think and act. When this change unfolds, we can then change how we participate in the world, becoming part of a critical mass through which the world itself can change (Johnson 2001; Rosen et al. 2017).

It is a common myth that healthcare providers are neutral observers treating clients and communities equitably no matter what they look like, what they believe, or how they act. Understanding the roots of our personal and collective bias can help move us to an understanding that all behaviors make sense in context and can lead us toward thinking and acting in ways that honor all diverse positions equally. Yet, it can prove challenging to identify and release familiar ways of thinking and acting to take a critical look at the ways we live that negatively impact the well-being of others. This may be particularly true for health professionals who have been rewarded for their expertise in professions with values and practices that differ sharply from those of many vulnerable clients and communities. In fact, inviting and integrating a foreign perspective is fundamentally unnatural, and when in the face of significant difference, discomfort, resistance and chaos are the most likely responses (Chang 2007; Fisher-Borne et al. 2015; Kai et al. 2007).

Pain, discomfort, and guilt around sensitive topics such as racism, ageism, sexism, ableism, heterosexism, and religious imperialism can generate resistance and dissuade healthcare providers from moving toward deeper self-awareness. At the same time, examining the development of prejudice and bias can be useful in helping providers move beyond the guilt or denial often associated with politically undesirable attitudes, to a deeper understanding of the societal influences that initiate and reinforce those ways of thinking. For example, healthcare providers not only address issues related to physical and mental health, but examine experiences related to discrimination, power and privilege, adaptation, strengths, and resilience. A perspective rooted in cultural humility consistently directs attention to social and political factors acknowledging the multidimensional nature of human experience that varies considerably within and across diverse and vulnerable groups (Fletcher 2015).

Developing self-awareness requires a safe context including self-compassion and a place for honest open dialogue with colleagues, clients, and communities. In addition, experiential learning activities can help healthcare providers imagine from multiple perspectives, reveal taken-for-granted assumptions, promote empathy toward alternate values, beliefs, and worldviews, and reveal areas for further reflection and understanding (Soulé 2019). When healthcare providers understand how their own values, beliefs, and worldviews have brought them to a specific viewpoint, or positionality, it is easier for them to understand the positionality or viewpoints of others. Consequently, a health professional can focus on developing self-awareness, working in collaboration with community members to assess healthcare systems, resource-sharing, alliance-building, priority setting, and collaborative problem solving while acknowledging the individuality and uniqueness of each client and their life-story. It can also mean recognizing the limits of our biomedical knowledge before the mystical nature of health and illness, and the profound wisdom and expertise of clients and their communities.

1.4 Leveling Power Differentials

Cultural humility focuses on the underlying systems that maintain power imbalances and keep structural disparities in place through recognizing and systematically analyzing these operations. Deepening awareness of the presence of privilege, a concurrent examination of how privilege operates, and the central role played by dominant groups in maintaining their place of privilege are needed to improve the quality of life for vulnerable populations. Privilege, a unique advantage that some individuals and groups have over others, includes enacting values of mainstream groups while suppressing or dismissing voices from non-mainstream groups. In a healthcare setting, this can include the role played by providers in influencing clients toward a biomedical model rather than organizing health system resources around clients' unique needs and priorities. Such a shift would transfer the responsibility for change from individual clients to the healthcare system itself. The current state of unbalanced power in healthcare interactions creates inequity in health outcomes among disparate groups, reinforces mistrust of healthcare providers and healthcare systems, and is not a context where optimal health can be achieved. Regrettably, vulnerable groups experience this power differential acutely while privileged groups often do not understand the impact of the privilege they hold, and in fact, their privilege may lie outside their conscious awareness. There is an urgent need for healthcare providers to become cognizant of their own place of privilege and accompanying power that exist because of specialized knowledge, professional and social rank, and socioeconomic status. Because only when aware of privilege, can providers then use this privilege to ally with those less privileged to eliminate health disparities and healthcare disparities. Interacting from a starting point of self-awareness and humility rather than professional expertise generates a different type of healthcare encounter, one that is open to learn and collaborate with clients and communities for optimal health as they define it (Drevdahl et al. 2008; Hassouneh 2008).

1.5   Building High-Quality Partnerships

A starting point for building high-quality partnerships is an understanding that individuals and groups brought up in widely varying contexts and backgrounds live in widely different realities or truths. To understand the lived experience of others, we must first have self-awareness, and then attune intentionally to the experience of others, gaining clarity on client priorities and concerns in order to create an environment that fosters collaboration in negotiating a plan of care. Listening to understand, also referred to as attuned communication, is a state of being that allows us to access the lived worlds of others and is at the heart of feeling seen and understood. This connectivity builds trust and reassurance between provider and vulnerable client or community. Bearing witness to the experience of others and listening to understand their lived worlds can give us clues to their underlying concerns and well-being. Importantly, being seen and heard is, in and of itself, a profound and healing act. This meaningful human connection can bring about a sense of well-being for both client and healthcare provider and is the essence of high-quality, respectful partnerships (Seigel 2010). Listening to understand without competing agendas such as multitasking or attempting to inform, fix, or advise, supports and acknowledges the client as the expert in their own life, and therefore a collaborative partner in their own healing process. For the healthcare provider, it blends the role of expert and learner and works to reduce the power differential that is nearly always present in a healthcare encounter.

In contrast, vulnerable populations often exhibit fear and mistrust as they navigate US healthcare providers and systems. This fear and mistrust are well founded and not only rooted in previous personal experiences but also because of systematic oppression experienced by vulnerable communities over time. Therefore, to build equitable partnerships, healthcare providers and systems must acknowledge and take accountability for the ways each has contributed to the harm of vulnerable groups, and forge partnerships built on a balancing of power, eliciting and working from the priorities identified by members of vulnerable groups, and valuing diverse types of expertise and ways of knowing.

Empathy is the capacity to be aware of, sensitive to, and vicariously experience the feelings of others without having to communicate those understandings directly or verbally. Empathy is a virtue that is demonstrated in how we act toward and treat people more than something to be explained. While words have a role in expressing empathy, ultimately and more importantly, empathy is the ability to be receptive to others and effectively enter into their perceptual experience including intellectual, attitudinal, and behavioral aspects. Empathy builds trust, and individuals and communities who perceive healthcare providers as empathetic feel seen, understood, and valued. In contrast, healthcare providers with low levels of empathy are unable to accurately interpret what a client is feeling and therefore bypass or ignore what is most important to them (Webster 2010).

To create a different quality of conversation, healthcare providers can begin building trust by asking different kinds of questions than they typically have in the past. This will take both courage and a willingness to sit with discomfort. For example, providers can ask clients if they have had experiences where they have been treated poorly because of their dark skin, sexual orientation, or other dimensions of vulnerability they may possess. Providers can ask if that is something they are afraid will happen at this appointment, and if so, what can they do to help them feel comfortable. A provider's ability to ask such questions conveys something important— that they recognize that in the body that the client is in, they may have had experiences with healthcare providers or healthcare systems that have been difficult and painful, and that they may be worried they will have those experiences again. In fact, they may have had those experiences at their last appointment and may still be upset. A provider can reaffirm their willingness to listen and work with them to create a situation where it is less likely to happen again. And if it does, creating the possibility that they will have an ally to help them navigate the system, or at least to listen carefully and understand.

1.6 The Role of the Body in Developing Cultural Humility

An important distinction exists between cognitive and embodied knowing that shifts from knowing "about" vulnerable groups to an internal attunement "with" them. The division between mind and body—cognition and behavior—reinforces the current division in Western healthcare between the cognitive, affective, and behavioral aspects of experience. Yet it has long been known that values create a context that influences sensory perceptions, and that our bodies can be instruments to effectively gather information about others (Bennett and Castiglioni 2004; Damasio 1999; Langer 2001). An exclusive emphasis on the cognitive aspects of understanding can mask the deeper phenomenon of the embodiment of knowing others that can simplify and fragment the development of high-quality relationships. Because healthcare providers are in a practice that relies on developing perceptual acuities to see, hear, feel, and notice events and signs that they could not recognize before their education, understanding the physical nature of cultural humility can enhance perceptual abilities, discernment of patterns and distinctions, and nuances including empathy.

Importantly, when one of the primary foci in healthcare education and practice is cognitive knowing, implicitly the body including sensations and visceral responses are excluded as another important way of knowing. This exclusion of the body leads to a cognitive-based observation of experience rather than to the experience itself, which alienates us from the rich complexity of our physical experience (Horn and Wilburn 2005; Ludwig and Kabat-Zinn 2008). Knowledge alone is insufficient for successful engagement with others and it is also necessary to become sensitive to the *feelings* (multisensory awareness) that accompanies knowledge to build interpersonal connectivity (Dyche and Zayas 2001). This ability to physically experience one's own and another's experience is termed *embodiment*. When in familiar and comfortable settings, things simply "feel right." This *feeling right* can be considered the physical manifestation of ethnocentrism that perceives our own values, beliefs, and worldviews as central to reality. Furthermore, without a similar sense or *feeling* for vulnerable groups, we are limited in our depth of understanding and ability to adapt and build rapport with them (Bennett and Castiglioni 2004; Kim and Flaskerud 2007). Given the innate link between mind and body, anxiety, which is often present in the face of significant difference, is consistently accompanied by physical tension. Physiologically, this stricture of mind and body can lead to limited thinking and a skewing of perceptions, which may include withdrawal, defense, and/or hostility. These personal, often negative emotional reactions can either act as blocks to working effectively with vulnerable clients or become catalysts for further insight, self-awareness, and effective future interactions (Chang 2007).

1.7   Role of Cultural Humility in Healthcare Systems

There is no single solution to work effectively with vulnerable populations and each pairing of healthcare system and surrounding community will have a different set of unique priorities, challenges, strengths, and solutions. Understanding the distinctive priorities of specific communities can contribute to providing safe, quality care, decrease health disparities, and engage community in sharing their expertise, information, and resources. To create environments where cultural humility is the expected norm, a systems approach to developing institutional standards is required. Leadership can set a tone for integrating cultural humility throughout a healthcare system and can help to elevate the priority of cultural humility in all policies, drive systematic efforts, and inspire staff support. And while cultural humility is an important quality of client and community care, it is also necessary when building strong relations among a healthcare workforce that often includes large rank and class differences (Chrisman 2007).

Thinking and acting from a place of cultural humility is a transformational way to address the needs of vulnerable populations, increase work satisfaction, and build an inclusive healthcare environment where vulnerable individuals and communities feel safe, seen, heard, and valued. Cultural humility is a way of being in the world informed by a commitment to self-reflection and self-critique, becoming aware of and leveling power differentials, and building meaningful, authentic partnerships between client and healthcare provider, community, and healthcare system. While it can be challenging to learn to value different, even conflicting perspectives equally, the resulting meaningful connectivity serves both a local and global perspective. Staying curious, listening to understand, and remaining open-minded and open hearted can support healthcare providers to learn to sit comfortably in the tension of holding two or more disparate perspectives simultaneously and move us toward a more just and ethical world.

References

Abdul-Raheem J (2018) Cultural humility in nursing education. J Cult Divers 25(2):66–73

American Academy of Nursing (1992) The AAN expert panel on culturally competent nursing care. Nurs Outlook 40(6):277–283

American Nurses Associaetion (ANA) (2018) The nurse's role addressing discrimination: protecting and promoting inclusive strategies in practice settings, policy, and advocacy. www.nursingworld.org. Accessed 24 Jul 2020

Benner P, Sutphen N, Leonard V, Day L (2009) Educating nurses: a call for radical transformation. Jossey-Bass, San Francisco, CA

Bennett MJ, Castiglioni I (2004) Embodied ethnocentrism and the feeling of culture. In: Landis D, Bennett JM, Bennett MJ (eds) Handbook of intercultural training, 3rd edn. Sage, Thousand Oaks, CA

Betancourt JR, Maina AW (2004) The Institute of Medicine report "unequal treatment": implications for academic health centers. Mt Sinai J Med 71(5):314–321

Chang WW (2007) The negative can be positive for cultural competence. Hum Resour Dev Int 10(2):225–231

Chang E, Simon M, Dong X (2012) Integrating cultural humility into healthcare professional education and training. Adv Health Sci Educ 17:269–278

Chrisman NJ (2007) Extending cultural competence through systems change: academic, hospital, and community partnerships. J Transcult Nurs 18(1):68S–76S

Damasio A (1999) The feeling of what happens: body and emotion in the making of consciousness. Harcourt Brace, New York

de Chesnay M, Anderson BA (2016) Caring for the vulnerable. Jones & Bartlett Learning, Burlington, MA

Drevdahl DJ, Canales MK, Dorcy KS (2008) Of goldfish tanks and moonlight tricks: can cultural competence ameliorate health disparities? Adv Nurs Sci 31(1):13–27

Dunn A, Soulé I (2016) Cultural considerations for pediatric primary care, 6th edn. Elsevier, Amsterdam, pp 33–44

Dyche L, Zayas LH (2001) Cross-cultural empathy and training the contemporary psychotherapist. Clin Soc Work J 29(3):245–258

Fisher-Borne M, Cain JM, Martin SL (2015) From mastery to accountability: cultural humility as an alternative to cultural competence. Soc Work Educ 34(2):165–181

Fletcher SNE (2015) Cultural sensibility in healthcare. Sigma Theta Tau International, Indianapolis, IN

Gray DP, Thomas D (2005) Critical analysis of "culture" in nursing literature: implications for nursing education in the United States. Annu Rev Nurs Educ 3:249–270

Gregg J, Saha S (2006) Losing culture on the way to competence: the use and misuse of culture in medical education. Acad Med 81(6):542–547

Hassouneh D (2008) Reframing the diversity question: challenging Eurocentric power hierarchies in nursing education. J Nurs Educ 47(7):291–292

Horn J, Wilburn D (2005) The embodiment of learning. Educ Philos Theory 37(5):745–760

Institute of Medicine (IOM) (2003) In: Smedley BD, Stith AY, Nelson AR (eds) Committee on understanding and eliminating racial and ethnic disparities in health care. National Academies Press, Washington, DC

International Council of Nurses (ICN) (2018) Health of migrants, refugees and displaced persons. www.icn.ch. Accessed 24 Jul 2020

Johnson AG (2001) Privilege, power, and difference. McGraw Hill, Boston, MA

Kai J, Beavan J, Faull C, Dodson L, Gill P, Beighton A (2007) Professional uncertainty and disempowerment responding to ethnic diversity in healthcare: a qualitative study. Publ Libr Sci 4(11):e323

Kim S, Flaskerud JH (2007) Cultivating compassion across cultures. Issues Ment Health Nurs 28:931–934

Langer EJ (2001) Opening our minds to deepen our vision. PsycCRITIQUES 46(1):78–79

Ludwig DS, Kabat-Zinn J (2008) Mindfulness in medicine. JAMA 300(11):1350–1352

Masters C, Robinson D, Faulkner S, Patterson E, McIlraith T, Ansari A (2019) Addressing biases in patient care with the 5R's of cultural humility, a clinician teaching tool. J Gen Intern Med 34(4):627–630

Rosen D, McCall J, Goodkind S (2017) Teaching critical self-reflection through the lens of cultural humility: an assignment in a social work diversity course. Soc Work Educ 36(3):289–298

Seigel DJ (2010) Mindsight. Bantam, New York, NY

Soulé I (2019) The rule of 16: An experiential learning activity. J Nurs Educ 58(11):676. https://doi.org/10.3928/01484834-20191021-14.

Tervalon M, Murray-Garcia J (1998) Cultural humility versus cultural competence: a critical discussion in defining physician training outcomes in multicultural education. J Healthc Poor Underserved 9(2):117–125

Webster D (2010) Promoting empathy through a creative reflective teaching strategy: a mixed-method study. J Nurs Educ 49(2):87–94

World Health Organization (WHO) (2018) Social determinants of health. www.who.int. Accessed 24 Jul 2020

Addressing Health Inequities in Vulnerable Populations Through Social Justice

2

Layla J. Garrigues

2.1 Introduction

Understanding underlying root causes of what makes an individual, a group, community, or population of people vulnerable is vital in nursing practice. As nurses, we work with individuals and with groups whether they are families, caregivers, communities, or populations. In applying a social justice lens in nursing, we must consider the health inequities of vulnerable populations. Social justice is the underlying principle of population health nursing and a fundamental nursing value. The tenets of social justice require nurses to maintain and demonstrate health-related ethical, moral, humanitarian, and legal principles. Nursing practice is guided by the Nursing Code of Ethics which clearly outlines ethical obligations and duties nurses must follow in caring for vulnerable populations (American Nurses Association 2015).

2.2 Vulnerable Populations

Vulnerability definition: Vulnerability is the degree to which an individual or population is unable to anticipate, cope with, resist and recover from the impacts of negative or traumatic experiences (World Health Organization 2017). To be vulnerable means to be susceptible to negative events with little to no control over the effects of these events, often related to situational and social circumstances, environmental impacts, and unbalanced power and privilege. These negative experiences can be cumulative traumas resulting in chronic stress, comorbidity, and chronic illnesses. Or, they can also be temporary, acute vulnerability experienced by individuals or communities/populations.

L. J. Garrigues (✉)
School of Nursing, University of Portland, Portland, OR, USA
e-mail: garrigue@up.edu

© Springer Nature Switzerland AG 2021   11
A. Vermeesch (ed.), *Integrative Health Nursing Interventions for Vulnerable Populations*, https://doi.org/10.1007/978-3-030-60043-3_2

All people can be considered vulnerable at certain times due to their particular conditions in life. People can argue that vulnerability is just another label and consider that patronizing. To be sure, anyone can be vulnerable at any point in time given their circumstances. For example, nursing students and faculty can be considered vulnerable populations depending upon specific situations. Students transitioning from campuses back to the community in the middle of a semester due to a pandemic is not only unanticipated, but disruptive, anxiety-inducing, and challenging. In particular, the experience of underserved student populations during such a transition can be daunting can be daunting in addressing financial and housing needs, mental health services, and whether they have the ability to transfer or complete college.

Considerations include whether the vulnerability is situational and temporary or consistent and long-lasting. For example, healthcare providers who are also faculty are a vulnerable population during a pandemic working in conditions that expose them to highly virulent, infectious viruses.

Being vulnerable is a state of defenselessness and fragility, the inability to withstand the disorder and disruptions of external and internal stressors, and being susceptible to harm (Aday 2001; Cardona 2004). It is the public health concept of risk at any given moment in time relative to other individuals or groups (Aday 2001). To be vulnerable means to have less control over one's health and to be at greater risk for illness or disability than others. This involves looking at comparative data between groups and populations. All countries have population groups who are more vulnerable to health threats than the general population.

People who are vulnerable are more likely to develop adverse health outcomes as a result of exposure to risk or to have worse outcomes from those health problems than the population as a whole (Aday 2001). Such people have less control over their health than the general population. They are more sensitive to risk factors because they are often exposed to cumulative risk factors and are more likely to suffer from health disparities. **Health disparities** are differences in health status between groups of people related to social, environmental, or demographic factors such as race, ethnicity, sexual orientation, income, or geographic region (Braveman et al. 2011; World Health Organization 2011).

Vulnerability results from the **combined effects (cumulative risks)** of limited physical, environmental, personal resources, and biopsychosocial resources. There is usually an interaction among the factors of poverty, housing, financial and social resources, environment, access to care, and family, physical, and emotional history. This situation is called **"allostatic load"** which is a phrase to describe the physiological consequences of chronic exposure to the fluctuating or heightened neural or neuroendocrine response that results from released or chronic stress (McEwen 2005). As a result, people and populations can have poor physical, social, or psychological health outcomes (Aday 2001). Major contributors for increased allostatic load are racist policies (systemic/structural/institutional racism) that cause populations to experience marginalization and chronic discrimination, and as a result, heightened stress hormones and chronic stress (Williams et al. 2019). The lack of a sense of control is related to privilege and power. Historical and structural inequities are the foundation for rendering certain populations in experiencing persistent marginalization and chronic vulnerability. An example is the state-sanctioned alienation from property and traditional lands taken from Native Americans—causing communities to live in poor housing conditions, lack of access to quality education, lack of jobs, poor services and infrastructure, and food insecurity (American Public Health Association 2018). Black Americans, even with higher incomes, experience greater and prolonged exposure to toxic pollutions than other populations, including white Americans with lower incomes (Smiley 2019). Being exposed to toxins over a lifetime causes increased morbidity and mortality (Smiley 2019; Ruiz et al. 2018).

An example of cumulative risks is the **Adverse Childhood Experiences (ACEs)**. The term "ACEs" originated from a study by the Centers for Disease Control and the Kaiser Permanente health care organization in California using data from over 17,000 members (CDC 2020). Although the original study was primarily of educated, upper-middle class, middle-aged white women, the study does provide valuable insights into the associations between ACEs and health outcomes. There have been further research studies looking at the different types of childhood adversities among other populations. The three specific types of adversity children faced in their home environment included various forms of physical and emotional abuse, neglect, and household dysfunction. Results of the study showed a strong correlation between the more ACEs experienced and the increased likelihood of poor health outcomes later in life, including chronic illnesses, increased risk of diabetes, heart disease, depression, smoking, substance abuse disorder, absenteeism from work and school, and increased mortality and morbidity (Center on the Developing Child, Harvard University 2020).

Familial trauma has adverse effects on populations. Black and Hispanic children and youth are more likely to experience ACEs than white and Asian children and youth. "To some extent, these racial disparities reflect the lasting effects of inequitable policies, practices, and social norms. Discriminatory housing and employment policies, bias in law enforcement and sentencing decisions, and immigration policies have concentrated disadvantage among black and Hispanic children, in particular, and leave them disproportionately vulnerable to traumatic experiences like ACEs" (para. 2) (Sachs and Murphey 2018).

Vulnerable populations often experience **multiple cumulative risks** such as environmental hazards (e.g., exposure to harsh conditions, toxins, or communicable diseases), place of residence (e.g., unstable housing), social hazards (e.g., exposure to systemic, structural, and/or institutional racism), health status (e.g., comorbid conditions such as diabetes and depression), poverty and financial circumstances, personal behaviors/characteristics and lifestyle (e.g., smoking, vaping, sedentary lifestyle, internal sense of control such as lack of motivation, low self-esteem, or learned helplessness related to lack of control), biological or genetic makeup (e.g. hormones, changes in normal physiology), livelihood, cultural beliefs, age, sexual orientation, functional or developmental status, ability to communicate effectively, race, and ethnicity.

These cumulative risks can be categorized as **internal and external factors** making a person or population susceptible to poor health outcomes. Vulnerability results from the interaction of internal and external factors (Appleton 1994). Internal factors include personal coping skills, attitudes, beliefs, and behaviors. External factors include the environment, policies, and social capital (the networks of relationships among people who live and work in a particular society, enabling that society to function effectively). Social capitals are the value and benefits that comes from social relationships and networks (Putnam 2004).

Vulnerability can be analyzed at **two levels**, (1) on an individual level (looking at each person) or (2) at an aggregate level (which looks at the whole formed by combining several, typically disparate, elements) such as looking at a community or a population. Most of the literature looks at vulnerability at the aggregate view of vulnerable populations. Some common **health statistics** include incidence which is the number of new cases, prevalence is the number of cases of a disease at a given time, mortality rate (the number of deaths in a certain group of people during a certain time period), and survival rate (the length of survival following diagnosis). Morbidity refers to the presence of disease or symptoms of a disease within a group of people. **Relative risk** is a "ratio of the probability of an event occurring in the exposed group versus the probability of the event occurring in the non-exposed group" (para. 1) (Tenny and Hoffman 2020). A **risk factor** is "any attribute, characteristic or exposure of an individual that increases the likelihood of developing a disease or injury" (para. 1) (World Health Organization 2019). Some examples of **risk factors** include malnutrition, unsafe sex, hypertension, exposure to toxic air or water pollution, and drug and alcohol abuse.

Poverty is a growing problem in the U.S. with a widening gap between extreme wealth and extreme poverty (Chokshi 2018). Clearly, **poverty** and low socioeconomic status are major contributors to **vulnerability**. People with low income are more likely to live and work in areas exposed to potential hazards, and less likely to have the resources to cope when a disaster strikes. Health effects of poverty include an increased mortality and morbidity due to racism, gender inequalities, poor housing, neighborhood violence, poverty stressors, educational and job status. People with low income have higher rates of chronic illnesses and infant morbidity and mortality, shorter life expectancy, and more complex health problems. Our current healthcare and social service systems are disjointed and fragmented in attempting to support people who are marginalized. Family dysfunctions and loss of support can result in social isolation and further lack of resources, continuing the spiral of poverty and increasing vulnerability, marginalization, and disenfranchisement (Wilson and Neville 2008; Baah et al. 2019).

Examples of vulnerable populations include those who have comorbid conditions or illnesses such as severe mental illness, compromised immune systems, substance use disorders, those who have experienced violence and trauma, economically disadvantaged, houseless, LGBTQIA+ populations, communities within urban areas and isolated rural locations with limited or no access to care, prisoners/ex-convicts, racial and ethnic minorities, uninsured, veterans, older adults, pregnant adolescents, low-income children, immigrants, refugees, and asylees. Vulnerable populations may not have the finances or insurance coverage to access care or navigate through the complex health system. Psychosocial trauma such as intergenerational trauma from suppressive policies and racism can cause chronic illnesses and shorter lifespans of marginalized populations.

Health care access example: Some issues around **reduced access** to care can include lack of transportation, inability to leave jobs for appointments, lack of health insurance, long waiting periods to access Medicaid coverage, no sick time coverage granted from work, unequal care, inconsistent care, treatment without health promotion, limited healthcare providers, and limited health/social resources. In addition to challenges accessing healthcare, clients can experience frustrations related to negative condescending attitudes by healthcare providers and issues around lack of health literacy. For example, using medical terminology that clients do not understand, ineffective translation or explanation of discharge instructions from inpatient settings, and medication labels in a language that clients may not comprehend. All of these health care access and experience issues are preventable given sufficient national attention and funding and should be addressed for health equity.

2.3   Social Justice

The concept of vulnerability involves social justice, equity, health equity, health inequities, health disparities, social determinants of health (SDOH), −isms, biases, cultural humility, and the difference between equality and equity.

2.3.1   Determinants of Health

The overarching goals of Healthy People 2030 sets the national agenda for addressing determinants of health of vulnerable populations, improving health and achieving health equity. These evidence-based goals include to "attain healthy, thriving lives and well-being, free of preventable disease, disability, injury and premature death. Eliminate health disparities, achieve health equity, and attain health literacy to improve the health and well-being of all. Create social, physical, and economic environments that promote attaining full potential for health and well-being for all. Promote healthy development, healthy behaviors and well-being across all life stages" (U.S. Department of Health and Human Services 2020) And finally, to "engage leadership, key constituents, and the public across multiple sectors to take action and design policies that improve the health and well-being of all" (para. 9) (U.S. Department of Health and Human Services 2020).

These Healthy People 2030 overarching goals apply to healthcare providers in their work to eliminate avoidable health inequities and disparities by attending to the most vulnerable groups. This involves addressing preventative measures which includes (1) **Primary prevention**: **Health promotion** or increased control over health which involves promoting health prior to disease or injury such as health policies for providing prenatal healthcare. These promotive practices rally healthy behaviors and support self-defined goals of clients and not the personal goals of the healthcare providers, (2) **Secondary prevention**: Detecting disease in early stages such as free or low-cost screenings. These are supportive healthcare practices aimed to modify any probable healthcare issues from worsening, and (3) **Tertiary prevention**: Rehabilitation or treatment such as insulin and glucometer strips at low cost for vulnerable populations. These are restorative practices aimed to adjust or alter adverse health outcomes. To tend to health inequities and disparities we need to understand determinants of health and impacts on populations. Nurses can help clients establish a primary care provider at a medical home, advocate for children and adults with behavioral health issues to receive appropriate and timely care, address primary prevention to reduce asthma-related deaths, and address risks for sexually transmitted infections and teen pregnancies.

Determinants of health are factors known to influence and contribute to health. Determinants of health are the range of personal, social, economic, and environmental factors that influence health status (World Health Organization 2020). Determinants of health extend beyond healthcare sectors and include individual behaviors, biological and genetic determinants, and physical determinants. Examples of *individual behavior determinants* of health or personal health practices and coping skills include hand washing, physical activity, diet, and substance use. Examples of *biological* and *genetic determinants* of health include age, sex, family history of cardiac disease, and inherited conditions such as cystic fibrosis, sickle-cell anemia, and the increased risk for breast and ovarian cancer from BRCA1 or BRCA2 genes (U.S. Department of Health and Human Services 2014a). Examples of *physical determinants* include natural environment (e.g. weather patterns, climate change, vegetation), and built environment (e.g. buildings, neighborhoods, parks, schools, or transportation), exposure to toxic substances (e.g. from freeways, waste treatment sites, factories, pesticides) (U.S. Department of Health and Human Services 2014a). Examples of *social determinants of health* (SDOH) include social environment (e.g. exposure to mass media, public safety, transportation options), social identity (e.g. job position, family/community positions), and social position (e.g. socioeconomic conditions, poverty, residential segregation) (U.S. Department of Health and Human Services 2014a).

These determinants of health, beyond the healthcare sector, are important in contributing to improving health of populations (U.S. Department of Health and Human Services 2014a). All of these are influenced by policies which impact the health of populations—whether benefiting some and hindering others. It is a continuous balancing act that needs careful scrutiny and attention in ensuring vulnerable populations are not further marginalized.

2.3.2 Health Disparities

Health disparity refers to a higher burden of illness, injury, disability, or mortality experienced by one group relative to another. For example, **oral health disparity** among certain populations includes methamphetamine abuse resulting in poor oral health. Health Disparities are **differences in health outcomes** between population groups. Health disparities mean the same thing as **health inequalities**. They are *differences* in the presence of disease, health outcomes, or access to health care between population groups. A health disparity occurs when there is a discrepancy between populations where one population has a higher incidence of an illness, higher mortality rate, or shorter survival time than another population. Both prevalence and incidence rates are considered when evaluating health disparities (Dye et al. 2019).

An example of health disparity can be seen in education. Early dropout rate from school is associated with poor health outcomes such as inadequate nutritional intake and choices, sedentary lifestyle, substance use disorder, social adjustment issues, teenage pregnancy, and shorter life spans when compared to people who have more education (CDC 2018). Some of these preventable issues stem from unequal opportunities, lack of funding, teacher quality and salaries, class sizes, and social and environmental distractions.

Natural health differences that occur from hormones or menopause, or basic biological differences not related to discrimination can be considered health disparities, but are not considered health inequities. If a disparity is determined to be *unfair and avoidable*, then it is considered an inequity (Carter-Pokras and Baquet 2002).

2.3.3 Health Inequities

Equity does not mean equality. Equity means fairness and addresses that everybody gets "the something" they *need*. **Equity** is a value judgment of what is fair. **Health equity** is the "attainment of the highest level of health for all people" (U.S. Department of Health and Human Services 2014b). And, beyond equity is inclusivity and justice, where traditionally marginalized and disenfranchised individuals' and communities' voices and opinions are honored, heard, and included in policy decision-making that impact their lives.

Social inequities reside in the structures of society, creating systematic differences in health outcomes between different population groups. Examples would include gender differences that arise from patriarchal norms or discrimination; class differences that arise from inequalities in wealth, power, and ownership and control of capital; and geographic differences that arise from higher exposures to risk or less access to remediable care or preventative resources (World Health Organization 2020). **Health inequities** refer to the differences in health that are unfair and unjust, and are *avoidable* (see Fig. 2.1). In Fig. 2.1, the proportions of the circles are illustrative and do not depict actual comparative data. Health inequities result from the impacts of socioeconomic status, environment, age, and various forms of discrimination such as gender, sexual identity, race, and ethnicity. Health inequities "adversely affect groups of people who have systematically experienced greater obstacles to health based on their racial or ethnic group; religion; socioeconomic status; gender; age; mental health; cognitive, sensory, or physical disability; sexual orientation or gender identity; geographic location; or other characteristics historically linked to discrimination or exclusion" (U.S. Department of Health and Human Services 2014b).

Fig. 2.1 Health disparities
and health inequities

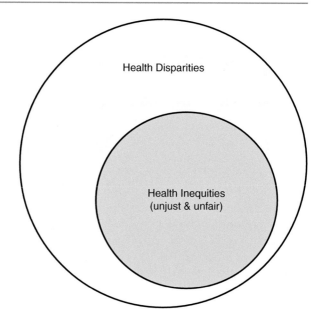

2.4   Systemic Racism

In addressing social inequities of vulnerable populations it is vital to understand the generational impacts of systemic racism which involves institutional, legalized racial discrimination (Jones 2001) such as unfair distributions, prohibitions in owning land, preventing home ownership (e.g., redlining), and the inability to vote. "Institutional racism in one sector reinforces it in other sectors, forming a large, interconnected system of structural racism whereby unfair discriminatory practices and inequities in the health and criminal justice systems and in labor and housing markets bolster unfair discriminatory practices and inequities in the educational system, and vice versa" (p. 1454) (Bailey et al. 2017). Structural, institutional, and systemic racism are functionally all the same—they all boil down to racist policies (Kendi 2019).

Concept of "Race": In order to address the issue of racism it is necessary to first understand the arbitrary nature of the very concept of "race." The concept of "race" is a social construct that is used to categorize and divide people based on physical characteristics (Fletcher 2015). Individuals can be of the same "race" but have different cultures. There are no alleles for "race." Rather, there are phenotypes which are the physical expression, or characteristics, of a trait. The interaction between phenotypes and genotypes is exceptionally complicated—not all phenotypic traits are expressed due to latent, inhibited, or recessive genes (Pierce 2006). Race is sometimes thought of in biological terms (for some people, it has biological meaning) based on the belief that there exist hereditary physical differences among people that define membership in a particular group. However, there are no measurable genetic characteristics that distinguish one group of people from another, in fact, there are more genetic differences among people who are labeled "Black" than there are differences between

"Blacks" and people labeled "White." In other words, there are often more genetic similarities between a Black person and a white person than between two Black people (Witherspoon et al. 2007). Although the concept of "race" does "not have a biological meaning, it does have a social meaning which has been legally constructed" (pp. 6–7) (Haney Lopez 1994) with categorizations used for such things as the census data and the Centers for Disease Control and Prevention for data collection.

The health impact of unjust **health inequities** has adverse effects on populations causing social and economic deprivation. For example, babies born to Black women are more likely to die during their first year of life compared to babies born to White women—even when comparing with same income levels. This inequity can be linked to high levels of stress hormones from **systemic racism** experienced by the Black mothers resulting in premature death (NCHS 2016). This is a health inequity and social and economic injustice because the difference between the populations is avoidable, unjust, and unfair.

Nurses have the duty to strive to manage and overcome racism—on the unconscious and conscious individual level and at the system level. Nurses can knowingly strive to be an anti-racist which takes "persistent self-awareness, constant self-criticism, and regular self-examination" (Kendi 2019).

Biases, stereotypes, and prejudices: When caring for individuals, nurses need to treat each individual without stereotyping or prejudice. These are internal processes, the attitudes and beliefs that one holds: A **stereotype**, according to the sociological definition, is a fixed image or belief about a particular group of people (Fletcher 2015). **Bias** is the inclination to have skewed or one-sided views. Cultural bias is the process where we tend to judge other phenomena based on our own cultural preferences, or by the norms of a particular culture. For example, it is common cultural practice to take off one's shoes before entering homes in some Asian countries such as Japan and South Korea, but not standard practice in some European countries or Western influenced cultures, although this is changing as practices and cultural beliefs evolve and change over time. **Cultural clashing** is an issue that can occur between and among healthcare providers and clients. This is when individuals or groups have opposing cultures (values, beliefs, attitudes, behaviors, norms, and so on) toward a same issue, topic, or activity. For example, there is value judgment around how to eat food. Eating with clean hands is the preferred method for some cultures rather than using utensils. Some cultures may deem the habit of eating with hands as "unclean" or "primitive" while using a spoon or fork as "natural and hygienic." Consider how cooks often prepare food with bare hands in the kitchen. Also consider how you might not know how the utensils are cleansed at a restaurant versus your personal knowledge about the cleanliness of your own hands. Using clean hands and clean utensils are both valid and useful means for eating food—nurses need to understand and advocate for their client's preferred method while also balancing client safety. **Prejudice** is an unjustified, incorrect, and "disapproving or negative attitude that is not rooted in fact or accurate information" about a concept, person, or group of people (p. 101) (Fletcher 2015). For example, a healthcare provider may have transphobia and may be uncomfortable, inattentive, and provide inappropriate care for their transgender client.

Discrimination is the behavior or actions based on prejudicial beliefs or attitudes, usually negative, toward an individual or group of people, such as on the basis on race, culture, gender, sexual orientation, able bodiedness, size, etc. These are the -isms that one holds against an individual or group. For example, Black patients significantly received less pain medications in the emergency room compared to White clients (57% vs. 74%), despite having similar reports of pain for their fractures (Todd et al. 2000). This is attributed to the inaccurate belief that Blacks feel less pain along with healthcare providers' prejudice and biases (Hoffman et al. 2016).

Ethnocentrism is a concept where people judge others' behaviors and beliefs by the norms of their own culture, and they consider their own culture to be superior to that of the other. For example, someone may have the belief that the only way to treat people is by using Western medicine and not considering other modalities, cultural approaches, and integrative health approaches, as valid or useful. This value judgment was previously described regarding eating with bare hands versus using utensils.

2.5   Taking Action: What Can Nurses Do?

2.5.1   Wellness Strategies as Part of Social Justice in Addressing Health Inequities

Nurses practicing cultural humility can best support clients by having self-awareness of their own biases, prejudices, and stereotypes while working with vulnerable populations. Care for vulnerable populations needs to be delivered by multidisciplinary teams focused on prevention, self-management, advocacy, and empowerment of individuals and communities/populations. Nurses, in collaboration with interprofessional teams can address and dismantle structural barriers for vulnerable populations. To confront these barriers, we can visualize three components in what we can call the nursing sphere of action in addressing health inequities (see Fig. 2.2). Although a reiterative and nonlinear process, the figure shows the components

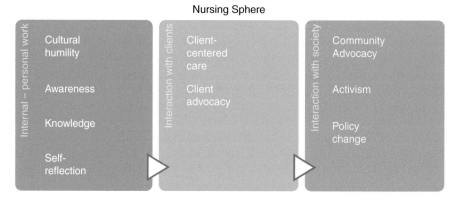

Fig. 2.2 Nursing sphere of action

proceeding from internal-personal work, to interaction with clients, to the wider sphere of interacting with society.

Cultural humility was explored in Chap. 1 and is the recognition of the limitations of one's own cultural perspective coupled with the lifetime work of overcoming biases, prejudices, and stereotypes in order to provide better nursing care to all clients (Fletcher 2015). This is the **internal, personal work** of each nurse in their practice of cultural humility, self-awareness, knowledge, and self-reflection (see Fig. 2.2). **Cultural competence** comprises of four components: (a) Awareness of one's own cultural worldview, (b) Attitude toward cultural differences, (c) Knowledge of different cultural practices and worldviews, and (d) cross-cultural skills (Martin and Vaughn 2007). Cultural competence in providing client-centered care is a process and involves life-long, ongoing learning as we can never be completely culturally competent since cultures are vast, continuously morphing, adapting, and changing, and have individual nuances as well.

Addressing Personal Biases: Bracketing is an approach that healthcare providers can use for addressing their own biases, stereotypes, and prejudices while working with clients (Fletcher 2015). This process addresses the internal thought processes, oftentimes unconscious, focuses on making them explicit and conscious, active listening and understanding disenfranchised voices, and attempts to address the discriminatory behavior or actions that can occur as a result of negative and inaccurate beliefs about a person, group, or population. This approach is an intentional self-reflection activity where a person consciously identifies their biases, preconceptions, judgements, beliefs, assumptions, knowledge, and experiences about a certain situation or encounter. The person acknowledges their own biases and prejudices they may hold and work to address them in a logical manner, while keeping themselves in check when providing the best possible unbiased care for their clients. Bracketing is only part of the work in addressing implicit biases and prejudices. Continuous self-scrutiny is a deliberate effort for a life-long and evaluative process that is part of cultural humility and cultural sensibility.

Nurses also **interact with their clients**, focusing on client-centered care and client advocacy (see Fig. 2.2). Nurses can advocate for the use of cultural practices that are not harmful for their clients. It is not about treating everyone equally, rather it is about addressing each client's unique healthcare and personal cultural needs. "If we have to tilt programs to meet the needs of one group in a different way than others, that would be…providing equity" (p. 497) (Pauly et al. 2017). **Resource Availability:** Healthcare providers need to assess their clients regarding resources available to individuals and populations. This includes societal and environmental resources (protective factors) such as social support. A recently published survey finds that about one in four hospitals and one in six physician practices screen their clients for social determinants of health (the social conditions that affect health, such as food access, housing stability, utility and transportation needs, and interpersonal violence) (Fraze et al. 2019). How can a healthcare provider improve screening for determinants of health? Some examples include questioning clients about their access to nutritious food, adequate and safe housing, available transportation to resources and healthcare, financial ability to pay for medications, supplies (e.g., insulin syringes), durable medical equipment, financial ability to pay for utilities and housing (whether mortgage payments or rent), and caregiver needs including respite care.

Finally, nurses **interact with society** that can involve community advocacy, activism, and policy change (see Fig. 2.2). Let us explore the intersection of **social justice and nursing**: Social justice implies that there is a fair and equitable distribution of benefits and burdens in a society. Social justice in action involves the process by which people work together at the local or community level to increase the power or control they have over the events and outcomes that has influence on all levels of their lives. On an individual level, this involves viewing situations as surmountable challenges and approaching with strength and resilience, but there needs to be the capacity making lasting changes in policies and laws. When working with vulnerable populations, nurses can **advocate** for them in many different ways—oftentimes helping clients/populations break out of the cycle of vulnerability.

Advocating for Policy Change: Eliminating avoidable health inequities and disparities cannot be accomplished without seriously addressing the underlying social determinants of health, many of which are shaped and perpetuated by bias, injustice and inequity (Braveman et al. 2011). We can work to eliminate avoidable health inequities and disparities by attending to most vulnerable groups.

According to the ANA Code of Ethics, "Advocacy is the act or process of pleading for, supporting, or recommending a cause or course of action. Advocacy may be for persons (whether as an individual, group, population, or society) or for an issue, such as potable water or global health" (p. 41) (American Nurses Association 2015). Advocacy can be done on an individual level or larger scale for instance, with policy change. This involves addressing political exclusion of certain populations and communities, investigating health-related burdens of healthcare cost and illness- and injury-related morbidity and mortality, and addressing such things as access to high quality prenatal care, clean air and water, and healthcare providers who use cultural humility and sensibility in working with their clients (World Health Organization 2011). Community empowerment may include community participation, hearing from disenfranchised and marginalized voices, community member leadership, changes to organizational structures, problem assessments at the grassroots level, mobilization of resources for those who need it the most, inquiring and questioning things, connecting with and collaborating with others such as outside agents and organizations, and program management (Minnesota Department of Health 2019). According to the ANA Code of Ethics, nurses should take socially just actions targeted at balancing health-related benefits and burdens for all members of society no matter their background, race, ethnicity, religion, age, etc. This is a vital duty of nurses in providing equitable and socially just care.

2.6   Conclusion

All countries have population groups who are more vulnerable to health threats than the general population. Nurses have the ethical duty to provide equitable, socially just care for clients whether individuals, groups, or communities, and to ensure the healthcare systems are equitable to promote autonomy, inclusive engagement, and preserve cultural safety for the prosperity of vulnerable populations in society (American Nurses Association 2015; Clark and Preto 2018). According to the American Nurses Association, 2015, it is imperative for vulnerable populations to receive special protection which is part of justice. This includes populations with behavioral health problems, learning disabilities, and any marginalized and disenfranchised populations (American Nurses Association 2015). Nursing innovations can range from quality-improvement projects at a unit-wide scale, to community level projects or organizations, to large scale policy change at the state and federal levels. For example, nurses led an innovative change to decrease the incidence of ventilator-associated pneumonia by changing the practice of elevating the head of the bed for patients, thereby improving patient health outcomes and reducing costs (Grap et al. 2005). Another nursing research investigated the importance of telehealth in various settings, advocating for change and innovation to reach marginalized populations (Grady 2014). During a pandemic causing disproportionate burden of illness and death among racial and ethnic groups, nurses are using telehealth to provide outreach and tele-triage as a means to address the health disparity experienced by vulnerable populations. From a public health perspective, nurses have a responsibility to address biases and -isms, in particular racism, and to lobby to improve policy, legislation, and practice to ensure marginalized and disenfranchised vulnerable populations receive health equity, and are empowered to voice their autonomy.

References

Aday L (2001) At risk in America. Jossey-Bass, San Francisco, CA

American Nurses Association (2015) Code of ethics for nurses with interpretive statements. Nursesbooks.org, Silver Spring, MD

American Public Health Association (2018) Priorities in tribal public health. https://www.apha.org/-/media/files/pdf/topics/environment/partners/tpeh/priorities_tribal_health_2018.ashx?la=en&hash=C06951A62A5E215BE6C99442A9E1E9DDD060B7C6. Accessed 20 Jul 2020

Appleton JV (1994) The concept of vulnerability in relation to child protection: health visitors' perceptions. J Adv Nurs 20:1132–1140. https://doi.org/10.1046/j.1365-2648.1994.20061132.x

Baah FO, Teitelman AM, Riegel B (2019) Marginalization: conceptualizing patient vulnerabilities in the framework of social determinants of health: an integrative review. Nurs Inq 26(1):e12268. https://doi.org/10.1111/nin.12268

Bailey Z, Krieger N, Agénor M, Graves J, Linos N, Bassett M (2017) Structural racism and health inequities in the USA: evidence and interventions. Lancet 389:1453–1463. https://doi.org/10.1016/S0140-6736(17)30569-X

Braveman PA, Kumanyika S, Fielding J, Laveist T, Borrell LN, Manderscheid R et al (2011) Health disparities and health equity: the issue is justice. Am J Public Health 101(Suppl 1):S149–S155. https://doi.org/10.2105/AJPH.2010.300062

Cardona OD (2004) The need for rethinking the concepts of vulnerability and risk from a holistic perspective: a necessary review and criticism for effective risk management. In: Bankoff G, Frerks G, Hilhorst D (eds) Mapping vulnerability: disasters, development and people. Earthscan, London, pp 37–51

Carter-Pokras O, Baquet C (2002) What is a "health disparity"? Public Health Rep 117(5):426–434. https://doi.org/10.1093/phr/117.5.426

CDC (2018) Health disparities. https://www.cdc.gov/healthyyouth/disparities/index.htm. Accessed 31 May 2020

CDC (2020) About the CDC-Kaiser ACE Study. https://www.cdc.gov/violenceprevention/childabuseandneglect/acestudy/about.html. Accessed 20 Jul 2020

Center on the Developing Child, Harvard University (2020) ACEs and toxic stress: frequently asked questions. https://developingchild.harvard.edu/resources/aces-and-toxic-stress-frequently-asked-questions/. Accessed 12 Jul 2020

Clark B, Preto N. Exploring the concept of vulnerability in health care. CMAJ. 2018;190:E309–9. https://doi.org/10.1503/cmaj.180242

Chokshi DA (2018) Income, poverty, and health inequality. JAMA 319:1312–1313. https://doi.org/10.1001/jama.2018.2521

Dye BA, Duran DG, Murray DM, Creswell JW, Richard P, Farhat T et al (2019) The importance of evaluating health disparities research. Am J Public Health 109(S1):S34–S40. https://doi.org/10.2105/AJPH.2018.304808

Fletcher SNE (2015) Cultural sensibility in healthcare: a personal & professional guidebook. Sigma Theta Tau International, ProQuest Ebook Central, Indianapolis, IN

Fraze TK, Brewster AL, Lewis VA (2019) Prevalence of screening for food insecurity, housing instability, utility needs, transportation needs, and interpersonal violence by us physician practices and hospitals. JAMA Netw Open 2:e1911514. PMCID: PMC6752088. https://doi.org/10.1001/jamanetworkopen.2019.11514

Grady J (2014) Telehealth: a care study in disruptive innovation. Am J Nurs 114:38–45. https://doi.org/10.1097/01.NAJ.0000445682.52553.89

Grap MJ, Munro CL, Hummel RS, Elswick RK, McKinney JL, Sessler CN (2005) Effect of backrest elevation on the development of ventilator-associated pneumonia. Am J Crit Care 14:325–332

Haney Lopez IF (1994) The social construction of race: some observations on illusion, fabrication, and choice. Harv Civil Rights Civil Liber Law Rev 29:1–62. 6–7, 11–17

Hoffman KM, Trawalter S, Axt JR, Oliver MN (2016) Racial bias in pain assessment and treatment recommendations, and false beliefs about biological differences between blacks and whites. Proc Natl Acad Sci 113:4296–4301. https://doi.org/10.1073/pnas.1516047113

Jones C (2001) Levels of racism: a theoretic framework and a gardener's tale. Am J Public Health 90:1212–1215. https://doi.org/10.2105/ajph.90.8.1212

Kendi IX (2019) How to be an antiracist, 1st edn. One World, New York

Martin M, Vaughn BE (2007) Strategic diversity & inclusion management magazine. DTUI Publications Division, San Francisco, pp 31–36

McEwen BS (2005) Stressed or stressed out: what is the difference? J Psychiatry Neurosci 30:315–318

Minnesota Department of Health (2019) Public health interventions: applications for public health nursing practice, 2nd edn. Minnesota Department of Health, St Paul, MN

NCHS (2016) Health, United States, 2015: with special feature on racial and ethnic health disparities. National Center for Health Statistics, Hyattsville, MD

Pauly BM, Shahram SZ, Dang P, Marcellus L, MacDonald M (2017) Health equity talk: understandings of health equity among health leaders. AIMS Publ Health 4:490–512. https://doi.org/10.3934/publichealth.2017.5.490

Pierce B (2006) Genetics: a conceptual approach, 2nd edn. W. H. Freeman, New York

Putnam RD (2004) Health by association: some comments. Int J Epidemiol 33:667–671

Ruiz D, Becerra M, Jagai JS, Ard K, Sargis RM (2018) Disparities in environmental exposures to endocrine-disrupting chemicals and diabetes risk in vulnerable populations. Diabetes Care 41:193–205. https://doi.org/10.2337/dc16-2765

Sachs V, Murphey D (2018) The prevalence of adverse childhood experiences, nationally, by state, and by race or ethnicity. Child trends. https://www.childtrends.org/publications/prevalence-adverse-childhood-experiences-nationally-state-race-ethnicity. Accessed 12 Jul 2020

Smiley K (2019) Racial and environmental inequalities in spatial patterns in asthma prevalence in the US south. Southeast Geogr 59:389–402. https://doi.org/10.1353/sgo.2019.0031

Tenny S, Hoffman MR (2020) Relative risk. Treasure Island, FL: StatPearls. https://www.ncbi.nlm.nih.gov/books/NBK430824/. Accessed 12 Jul 2020

Todd KH, Deaton C, D'Adamo AP, Goe L (2000) Ethnicity and analgesic practice. Ann Emerg Med 35:11–16. https://doi.org/10.1016/s0196-0644(00)70099-0

U.S. Department of Health and Human Services (2014a) Determinants of health. https://www.healthypeople.gov/2020/about/foundation-health-measures/Determinants-of-Health. Accessed 28 Jul 2020

U.S. Department of Health and Human Services (2014b) Disparities. https://www.healthypeople.gov/2020/about/foundation-health-measures/Disparities. Accessed 28 Jul 2020

U.S. Department of Health and Human Services (2020) Healthy People 2030 Framework. https://www.healthypeople.gov/2020/About-Healthy-People/Development-Healthy-People-2030/Framework. Accessed 28 Jul 2020

Williams DR, Lawrence JA, Davis BA, Vu C (2019) Understanding how discrimination can affect health. Health Serv Res 54(Suppl 2):1374–1388. https://doi.org/10.1111/1475-6773.13222

Wilson D, Neville S (2008) Nursing their way not our way: working with vulnerable and marginalized populations. Contemp Nurse 27:165–176. https://doi.org/10.5555/conu.2008.27.2.165

Witherspoon DJ, Wooding S, Rogers AR, Marchani EE, Watkins WS, Batzer MA, Jorde LB (2007) Genetic similarities within and between human populations. Genetics 176:351–359. https://doi.org/10.1534/genetics.106.067355

World Health Organization (2011) A conceptual framework for action on the social determinants of health. https://www.who.int/social_determinants/corner/SDHDP2.pdf?ua=1. Accessed 20 Jul 2020

World Health Organization (2017) 10 facts on health inequities and their causes. https://www.who.int/features/factfiles/health_inequities/en/. Accessed 21 Jul 2020

World Health Organization (2019) Health topics: risk factors. https://www.who.int/gho/ncd/risk_factors/en/. Accessed 28 Jul 2020

World Health Organization (2020) Social determinants of health. https://www.who.int/social_determinants/en/. Accessed 28 Jul 2020

Resources

Compare levels of poverty between the states in the United States: Comparing Poverty Rates under the Official Census Poverty Measure and the Supplemental Poverty Measure: https://www.kff.org/interactive/seniors-in-poverty/. State profiles of women's health interactive map: https://www.kff.org/interactive/womens-health-profiles/?activeState=USA&activeCategoryIndex=0&activeView=map. https://www.kff.org/statedata/

Adverse Childhood Experiences (ACEs): Video: How childhood trauma affects health across a lifetime. Nadine Burke Harris, MD (CC) (15:59) https://www.ted.com/talks/nadine_burke_harris_how_childhood_trauma_affects_health_across_a_lifetime#t-602117

Health Equity: An example of health equity can be seen in tenant-based rental assistant programs such as this resource video by Dr. David Williams, Professor of Public Health, Harvard: https://www.youtube.com/watch?v=CwBEkGurMiY (4:17)

Explore how to achieve health equity is in the following video: Tools for a National Campaign Against Racism by Dr. Camara Jones, MD, MPH, PhD. https://www.youtube.com/watch?v=3aXoBfmSBNQ (1:16:38)

Implicit Association Test (IAT). The IAT measures the strength of associations between concepts (e.g., African American, Queer) and evaluations (e.g., good, bad) or stereotypes (e.g., athletic, clumsy). IAT results can change over time related to circumstances and how one has changed or adapted. The IAT test results are often best for aggregate results (looking at population group results such as within certain age range, etc.)

Resource Links

http://www.lookdifferent.org/what-can-i-do/implicit-association-test
https://implicit.harvard.edu/implicit/
https://larissapahomov.com/2015/12/09/teaching-bias-the-iat-test/

Integrative Health Interventions for the Vulnerable and Underserved

3

Pamela J. Potter

Integrative health and medicine utilize the best most efficacious and least invasive approaches for supporting health and wellness in individuals and populations. The Institute for Integrative Health distinguishes integrative medicine from integrative health. Integrative medicine focuses predominantly on clinical care, while "integrative health encompasses the full array of health determinants, including social, behavioral, economic, and environmental factors" (Witt 2017). People may choose complementary alternative integrative health (CAIH) modalities to complement the conventional medical care they receive. For consistency, the acronym CAIH will be used throughout this chapter, although articles reviewed may have used other acronyms to describe complementary, alternative, traditional, and integrative therapies or approaches to care (Pinzon-Perez 2016). Early research sought to determine who used these approaches, reasons for use, and communication with physicians; researchers were primarily concerned about safety and possible lack of compliance with conventional care. At first glance, statistics show CAIH approaches are used predominantly by white educated middle-class women (Bishop and Lewith 2010). Based on this data one might decide that such therapeutic approaches are not of interest to underserved and vulnerable populations. Or, if they are of interest, they are prohibitively expensive. Lack of knowledge may be a factor related to limited use of CAIH approaches by vulnerable populations. Understanding usage patterns is more complex. The premise of this chapter is that barriers due to structural racism must be considered when interpreting use of CAIH by underserved populations and when planning for CAIH interventions to support health and well-being of the vulnerable and underserved.

This chapter clarifies identification of CAIH intervention categories utilizing the Institute of Medicine (IOM) (2005) descriptors; defines vulnerable and underserved populations for this chapter; describes barriers to CAIH utilization; explores

P. J. Potter (✉)
School of Nursing, University of Portland, Portland, OR, USA

© Springer Nature Switzerland AG 2021   27
A. Vermeesch (ed.), *Integrative Health Nursing Interventions for Vulnerable Populations*, https://doi.org/10.1007/978-3-030-60043-3_3

reasons for nonuse and nondisclosure; identifies CAIH interventions used by vulnerable and underserved populations including use for specific health problems; reviews research on two CAIH modalities with specific populations; describes CAIH organizations that promote health in underserved and vulnerable populations; recommends approaches for increasing access and utilization of CAIH; and suggests nursing's role. This chapter focuses on CAIH use by vulnerable and underserved racial and ethnic groups, including CAIH use for conditions like cancer and diabetes. Salutogenic approaches for health like yoga and meditation provide examples of beneficial approaches to health promotion. This chapter does not address children, elderly, LGBTQ or specific diseases separate from racial and ethnic vulnerable populations.

3.1　Classifying CAIH Interventions

One way to organize CAIH interventions is to use an early classification described by the IOM (2005). This five-category classification structure includes: (1) Alternative medical systems, (2) Mind-body interventions, (3) Biologically based treatments, (4) Manipulative and body-based methods, and (5) Energy therapies. NCCIH currently uses three categories: Natural Products, Mind and Body Practices, and Other Complementary Approaches. These categories combine manipulative body-based therapies within Mind and Body practices, recategorize biology-based therapies under Natural Products, place alternative medical systems under Other Complementary Approaches, and minimally address energy therapies. Because of this limitation, the IOM categories will be used in this chapter (https://nccih.nih.gov/health/integrative-health#hed4).

Alternative medical systems refer to whole systems of medicine with theory and practice independent of conventional medicine (e.g. Ayurveda, Chinese Medicine, homeopathy, and naturopathy). A philosophical distinction between conventional biomedicine and traditional, complementary, alternative medical systems articulated by di Sarsina et al. (2012) observes that these systems of medicine understand health to encompass the whole person—inseparable body/psyche/spirit—while conventional medicine divides, localizes, and treats disease in various parts of the body.

Mind-body interventions include practices, based on the human mind, that influence the human body and physical health (e.g., biofeedback, hypnosis, meditation, prayer, tai chi, imagery, and yoga). Disease is not just something that happens to a person; the person has choice in how they respond. Popular among CAIH users, mind-body interventions are low cost, low risk (physical and emotional), and they empower the person to take an active role in their health (Wahbeh et al. 2008).

Biologically based therapies include specialized diets, herbal products, and other natural products such as minerals, hormones, and biologicals.

Manipulative and body-based methods include therapeutic approaches that incorporate movement or manipulation of the body (e.g., chiropractic, massage, Feldenkrais, Rolfing, among others).

Energy therapies include the manipulation and application of energy fields to the body. Some energy therapies involve external application of magnets or electronic devises. Energy therapies also include hands on energy healing applications (biofield therapies) like Reiki, qigong, Therapeutic Touch, and Healing Touch.

3.2   Who Are Vulnerable and Underserved Populations?

From the perspective of health, vulnerable populations consist of those communities and groups who—because of social, economic, and environmental barriers—experience poorer physical and mental health outcomes than the greater population (See Chap. 2 for more details). Vulnerable populations experience health disparities that can be observed and measured by comparing health outcomes among populations. Subjected to the stresses and social determinants of structural racism, Black and Hispanic populations demonstrate health disparities and experience the poorer health outcomes of vulnerable populations (Bailey et al. 2017). Access to and utilization of CAIH may also be subject to the structures in place that prevent racial/ethnic minorities from taking full advantage of the best approaches for supporting health and well-being. These considerations may be reflected in documentation of CAIH utilization surveys, conjectures about low utilization by racial/ethnic minorities, the creation of interventions designed for vulnerable and underserved populations, and the examination of the very structures of CAIH organizations.

3.3   Barriers to CAIH Utilization by Vulnerable Populations

Structural racism appears to be an underlying factor among the identified barriers to CAIH for the vulnerable and underserved. Saper (2016) identifies four barriers to CAIH use among the underserved: awareness, availability, accessibility, and affordability. **Awareness:** Populations with lower income, lower education, and lower literacy have lack of knowledge of these modalities. **Availability:** Similar to food deserts (areas with limited access to affordable healthy food options), CAIH provider establishments are less likely to be located in lower income areas. Mapping the availability of yoga studios, acupuncturists, and massage therapists in Boston, Saper's team found a minimal number of these providers in the low-income neighborhoods. **Accessibility:** Beyond awareness and availability, social determinants may impact the ability to utilize CAIH. Inflexible work schedules that cannot be adjusted to allow for attending classes, inefficient transportation that may be convoluted or expensive, inability to bring children or arrange for childcare, and language barriers impeding understanding contribute to limited accessibility. **Affordability:** Ability to pay for services not covered by insurance or provided as part of healthcare effectively limits choice of CAIH for low-income underserved people.

3.4   CAIH Use by Vulnerable Populations

Initial inquiries about the prevalence of CAIH use by the US population came from national surveys providing little insight into minority population use. Data mining of these surveys for utilization by specific populations (racial/ethnic or disease category) provides insights for further questions. In addition, regional studies with larger representation of the population of interests allow for greater understanding of CAIH use and qualitative focus group studies provide further insights on racial/ethnic minority populations.

Analyzing complementary health approaches the three National Health Interview Surveys (NHIS) conducted from 2002–2012, Clarke et al. (2015) reported an overall prevalence of CAIH use by 34% of adults in 2012. At this time, analysis providing an overall description of the 2017 NHIS data has not been published, although researchers are publishing findings on specific interventions like yoga and meditation. The ten most commonly used approaches include natural products (nonvitamin, nonmineral dietary supplements) (17.7%); deep breathing exercises (10.9%); yoga, tai chi, and qi gong (10.1%); chiropractic or osteopathic manipulation (8.4%), and meditation (8.0%), massage (6.9%), special diets (3.0%), homeopathy (2.2%), progressive relaxation (2.1%). Ayurveda, biofeedback, guided imagery, hypnosis, and energy healing therapy demonstrated a consistently low prevalence. Based on data thus far from these nationwide studies, Whites use a higher proportion of CAIH than minority populations. These global findings serve to reveal the divide between the White majority and ethnic minority CAIH use. Because the interest here is in utilization by underserved racial/ethnic minorities, those figures will be the primary focus. For uniformity and clarity, the terms Black, Hispanic, Asian, and White will generally be used when describing study findings.

3.4.1   Studies Targeting Use by Underserved Populations

Analysis of specific population subsets from the larger database studies provides a closer look at CAIH use by racial/ethnic minority populations.

Analysis of the 2002 NHIS data Black subset ($N = 4256$), when prayer for health (60%) was included as a variable, found that 67.6% used CAIH in the last 12 months, followed by herbals (14.2%) and relaxation (13.6%) (Brown et al. 2007). Users were more likely to be female, college educated, and insured. Treating specific health conditions, rather than prevention, was cited as the main reason for use.

Ward et al. (2013) conducted a systematic literature review of 36 original articles between 2002 and 2011 on the use of CAIH by Blacks. The majority of the articles reported 10% less use by Blacks, apart from prayer. The articles on specific health conditions tell another story of CAIH use by Blacks with diabetes, asthma, or anxiety (approximately 30% for some conditions). Interventions included herbal products, relaxation techniques, chiropractic, and acupuncture.

A study of Los Angeles county respondents ($N = 1044$) sought to compare CAIH utilization based upon two identical definitions with the exception that one included prayer as a variable (separate from spiritual healing) and the other excluded prayer (Robles et al. 2017). With prayer included 64% of the population reported CAIH use; without prayer 57% reported use. Higher income and women were more associated with use. With prayer included, significantly more of the Black population (79%) than Whites and all other populations used CAIH. Prayer (23%), massage (19%), megavitamins/supplements (14%), cleanse/fast (13%), and yoga (13%) comprised the highest use. Blacks and Whites showed highest use of megavitamins/dietary supplements (19% each), and Hispanics showed the highest use of cleanse/fasts (17%). Blacks and Hispanics showed the highest use of folk remedies (4% each).

Analysis of CAIH use, among a convenience sample of clients from a predominantly Hispanic community ($N = 150$, 74% Hispanic) at a clinic serving the medically underserved, found that 63% used at least one type of CAIH. The most commonly used were vitamins/supplements (32%), herbal medicine (29%), dietary/nutritional therapy (26%), massage (24%), meditation/relaxation (15%), and chiropractic (11%) (Ho et al. 2015). The presence of an Integrative Medicine residency at the clinic and a pilot Integrative Medicine consultation service possibly contributed to the positive comfort level of respondents. Although prior studies report that "60% of racial minorities do not disclose their CAM usage to their physicians" (p. 181), the majority were comfortable disclosing use to physicians, wanted to be asked about use, and thought physicians should be knowledgeable. They were interested in the introduction of massage, mind-body relaxation techniques, and acupuncture at the health center.

The Study of Women's Health Across the Nation, New Jersey site ($N = 171$, average age 61.8 years)—where respondents completed a general questionnaire and a culturally sensitive CAIH questionnaire designed to capture herbal products by Hispanic communities—demonstrated high use in both Hispanic (88.9%) and White women (81.3%) (Green et al. 2017). "Hispanic women were significantly less likely to consider herbal treatment [to be] drugs (16% vs. 37.5%; $p = 0.005$) and were less likely to report sharing the use of herbal remedies with their doctors (14.4% Hispanic vs. 34% non-Hispanic White; p = 0.001)" (p. 805). Botanicals, considered part of the Hispanic cultural tradition passed down by relatives, are seen as "naturally occurring remedies and part of common curative health practices in their countries of origin" (p. 309). Further, lack of health insurance and financial burden may contribute to choosing herbal preparations. The researchers also found few respondents reported use of self-help modalities like yoga. Cost and "cultural attitudes and spiritual beliefs toward yoga and other self-help modalities may result in lower use by some racial/ethnic groups" (p. 309).

3.4.2 Reasons for Nonuse

Lack of knowledge about CAIH is cited as a primary reason why minorities do not use these therapeutic approaches (Burke et al. 2015; Saper 2016). Some researchers speculate that low health literacy is the cause for lack of use, finding an association with low health literacy and lack of knowledge about CAIH. Although adequate health literacy in Whites is associated with increased use, and low health literacy is associated with lack of knowledge in Blacks, Blacks with adequate health literacy did not demonstrate increased CAIH use (Bains and Egede 2011). This suggests there may be other factors associated with lack of knowledge about CAIH. The history of Black and Hispanic populations with traditions of herbal and traditional medicine practices based on their cultural backgrounds, raises the speculation whether or not utilization research has been asking the right questions (Barnett et al. 2003). Research specifically directed at racial/ethnic minorities finds higher percentages of CAIH use where potential access is possible (Jones et al. 2018). Other identified factors influencing nonuse have previously been mentioned as barriers (awareness, availability, accessibility, and affordability).

3.4.3 Disclosure

National data studies previous research findings: Black, Hispanic, and Asian Americans are less likely to disclose CAIH use to healthcare providers compared to Whites (Chao et al. 2015). Compared to Whites, Blacks with access to high quality conventional care were more likely to discuss CAIH provider-based therapies with their medical providers rather than self-care therapies. Shelley et al. (2009) identified three themes that determine whether or not and how communication about CAIH takes place. Acceptance/nonjudgment by the clinician demonstrates an openness to discussion; the practitioner does not have to be an expert. Preferred initiation of communication by the practitioner; if the practitioner does not ask, discussion does not happen. Safety/efficacy concerns of the practitioner may result in a judgmental stance that inhibits communication. Further, assuming that no communication about CAIH means low use is an incorrect interpretation. Providers who take a patient-centeredness approach that asks open and nonjudgmental questions and adopt a participatory decision-making style are more likely to elicit patient disclosure of CAIH practices. Further, the presence of an Integrative Medicine residency contributes positively to patient comfort with disclosure (Ho et al. 2015).

3.4.4 Use for Specific Health Problems

3.4.4.1 Asthma

A survey conducted with parents ($N = 360$) of Vietnamese children with asthma reveals a 38.1% prevalence of parent-directed CAIH use (common therapies include steam inhalation, creams/topical oils, foods, prayer oil inhalation, massage, herbal medication, coining and cupping) (Berg et al. 2016). One reason for use included concern over long-term effects of conventional medication. In other studies, the researchers point out, CAIH use is not associated with nonadherence to conventional care, and actually, benefit has been demonstrated by some therapies (e.g., Chinese medicine). There are also serious dangers with the interaction of natural products and asthma medications (e.g., Natural Ephedra could potentiate albuterol) or the provocation of allergies (e.g., Echinacea and Chamomile are members of the ragweed family). The researchers recommend assessing for CAIH use to provide a more holistic approach to care.

3.4.4.2 Depression

A study of CAIH use in depressed underserved minority populations at a Los Angeles primary care clinic found over 57% of a sample of Black and Hispanic patients ($N = 315$) reported using CAIH (sometimes/often, 24%; frequently, 33%) (Bazargan et al. 2008). Lack of health insurance was the strongest predictor of use. Respondents reported use of biologically based approaches (58%), mind-body medicine (47%), manipulative and body-based practices (9%), and whole medical systems (8%). Black males demonstrating moderate depressive symptoms, no health insurance coverage, and higher self-rated health status were more likely to use CAIH for depression. The researchers conclude that underserved Blacks and Hispanics use CAIH to treat depression when conventional diagnosis and treatment access is limited.

Analysis of 2012 NHIS data on CAIH use from 6016 non-institutionalized adults with Moderate Mental Distress (MDD) (3492 Whites, 953 Blacks, 1078 Hispanics, 268 Asians, and 225 others) yielded estimates of specific CAIH prevalence related to race/ethnicity, sociodemographic, and health related factors (Rhee et al. 2016). The researchers found that CAIH use was higher among those with Moderate Mental Distress (40%) compared to those with less distress (32%). In adults with MMD, past year CAIH use differed significantly by race/ethnicity, ranging from 24.3% (Blacks) to 44.7% (Asians) and 46.8% (Others). Being younger, female, living in the West, higher education, being employed, more than four ambulatory care visits, and functional limitations were significantly associated with higher odds of CAIH use. Racial/ethnic differences appeared in the type of CAIH used. The "Other" group (American Indian, Alaska Native, and those reporting multiple races) used alternative medical systems, biologically based therapies, and energy therapies more than the other groups. Blacks reported least use of alternative medical systems, biologically based therapies, and manipulative body therapies. Hispanics reported least use of mind-body therapies and energy therapies. The data demonstrates use higher than the general population for persons with MDD. The researchers conclude that such knowledge could provide opportunities for communication among the varied providers (Conventional and CAIH) and integration of CAIH into care of people with MDD.

3.4.4.3 Cancer

Rush et al. (2016) conducted a study of Hispanic/Latina breast cancer survivors to learn CAIH use frequency and any associations with reported symptoms and functioning at baseline ($N = 136$) and over time (follow-up $n = 58$). Respondents reported using yoga, meditation, massage, or herbal/dietary supplements (35% baseline; 36% follow-up). A positive association with lower depression and better physical functioning and CAIH use was observed at baseline, while at follow-up CAIH use was associated with lower physical function and lower social role satisfaction. Devotional and spiritual practices at baseline predicted lower anxiety, depression, and fatigue in the follow-up group. Based on study findings, the researchers observe that CAIH "plays a complex and not always linear role in symptoms and function outcomes for Latina breast cancer survivors" (p. 1). Further, they suggest that the strong association between devotional and spiritual practices and reduced anxiety may inform anxiety-reduction interventions for this population.

A survey study of a medically underserved (MUPs) oncology patient population ($N = 169$) (43% Black, 28% Hispanic, 90% with income less than $10,000) assessed knowledge and use, deterrents to use, and interest/willingness to use CAIH (Jones et al. 2018). Respondents reported high use of prayer (85%), relaxation (54%), special diet (29%), meditation (19%), and massage (18%). Knowledge of CAIH was highest for prayer (97%) and lowest for herbs (60%). Hispanics (44.2%) and Blacks (69.2%) reported using relaxation techniques. Respondents expressed high level interest in prayer, massage, relaxation, herbal therapy, aromatherapy, special diet, meditation, yoga, and acupuncture if these were to be offered at the clinic. Identified barriers to CAIH use included lack of knowledge (21% acupuncture, 22% herb use) and cost (special diets, aromatherapy, herb use, massage, and yoga). Concluding that use and interest in CAIH is high among minority and medically underserved cancer population, the researchers stress the importance of professionally guided safe use.

3.4.4.4 Diabetes

As part of a Reducing Racial/Ethnic Disparities in Diabetes project, researchers at an academic medical center (Nguyen et al. 2014) conducted a survey of CAIH use by patients ($N = 410$) with type 2 diabetes. The study purpose was to compare sociodemographic and diabetes related factors in users and nonusers, to identify various modalities used by different ethnic groups, to determine influence of CAIH use on medication adherence, and to explore rationale for use. Vietnamese (57%) and Mexican Americans (53%) reported significantly more use in the past year than Whites (29%). Mexican Americans expressed more concern about diabetic complications, reported higher levels of nonadherence to medications because of cost, and demonstrated higher HbA1c values. Vietnamese Americans (47.1%) demonstrated higher use of CAIH practitioners compared to Mexican Americans (15.4%). Both Mexican (96.1%) and Vietnamese Americans (95.7%) reported high use of herbs and supplements. Mexican and Vietnamese Americans were significantly more likely to use CAIH instead of their diabetes medication ($p = 0.02$) than White respondents. Generally, the groups perceived CAIH to be more natural and to have fewer side effects than conventional medicine. Based on study findings, researchers stress the importance of communication about CAIH with underserved and vulnerable populations.

Desirous of learning about use of CAIH for weight loss and diabetes control by Hispanic women, Lindberg et al. (2019) conducted a survey of "alternative medicine, traditional Mexican medicine, and home remedies" used by Hispanic women ($N = 85$). Hispanic women demonstrate the highest estimated lifetime risk for diabetes among all genders and racial/ethnic groups, are less likely to achieve effective glycemic control, more likely to use "traditional" methods in addition to conventional medical care, and may be poorly informed about the best approaches for diabetes control. Part of an intervention study for diabetes management and risk reduction, the study group completed a survey of CAIH practices they used to control their diabetes and support weight management. Ninety-seven percent reported using at least one modality, with most respondents reporting not telling their provider. Those respondents ($n = 29$) with diabetes used personal attempts at diet modification (100%), home remedies (97%), herbs and teas (83%), licuado verde (green smoothie) (76%), exercise (69%), specific herbal products (41%), and massage by traditional healers for managing diabetic associated pain (20%). Most of the respondents with diabetes (86%) report "never" (58%) or "sometimes" (28%) disclosing CAIH use to their healthcare providers. Reflecting the lack of communication about CAIH use in light of potentially harmful as well as beneficial health consequences and the poor health outcomes associated with diabetes in Hispanic women, the researchers observe the importance of focusing on improved understanding and communication.

3.4.5 Specific Approaches: Meditation and Yoga

Analysis of the large database studies reveals an increasing trend in yoga and meditation practice by Blacks and Hispanics. Clarke et al. (2015) describe significant increases in use of yoga from 2002–2012 in both Hispanic (from 2.8% in 2002, 5.1% in 2012) and Black adults (2.5% in 2002, 5.6% in 2012). Examining the 2017 NIHS data on adult use of CAIH, Clarke et al. (2018) found yoga to be the most common for all respondents (9.3% in 2012, 14.3% in 2017). Hispanics (8.0%) and Blacks (9.3%) reported using yoga. Blacks (13.5%) reported higher use of meditation than Hispanics (10.9%). Significantly, these percentages suggest that an increasing utilization of yoga and meditation warrants consideration for enhancing the availability of these options for vulnerable populations.

Coughlin et al. (2015), identifying opportunities to address disparities in breast cancer survival and quality of life for Black women, describe CAIH approaches—mindfulness-based stress reduction and yoga—as interventions that have demonstrated benefit for breast cancer survivors. Reduced anxiety, depression, distress, and fatigue are among the possible benefits of yoga. Among cancer survivors, mindfulness-based stress reduction has demonstrated benefit for anxiety and depression. Intervention research on meditation and yoga provides opportunities to design culturally relevant interventions and learn about effectiveness with vulnerable populations.

3.4.5.1 Meditation

Underserved minority women breast cancer survivors receiving a 20-session contemplative self-healing intervention showed improved quality of life—with a clinically and statistically significant increase in the health-related quality of life and significant reduction in post-traumatic stress symptoms (Charlson et al. 2014).

Dresner et al. (2016) conducted a qualitative study of an 8-week medical group visit intervention for chronic pain patients ($n = 19$, 74% racial/ethnic minority). Visits included mindfulness-based stress (MBSR) reduction techniques (yoga, meditation, mindful eating, and body scan), education, and integrative medicine. Benefits included management of chronic pain and general health through self-regulation and mindfulness, diet and exercise, and self-monitoring.

Lyons et al. (2019) used an adaptation of the Mindfulness-Based Relapse Prevention curriculum for a 6-week intervention conducted within a drug treatment program at a large urban jail (Black, 58.9%; Hispanic, 18.6%). A culturally competent Black male with similar socioeconomic background as the detainees conducted the trainings. A small but significant increase in mindfulness was observed. The researchers found the intervention feasible in a jail setting and results suggested that it may facilitate reduction in drug craving and PTSD symptoms.

Correlating psychological stress with a negative impact on health, Woods-Giscombe et al. (2019) conducted a feasibility trial to compare an innovative MBSR program combined with diabetes risk reduction education ($n = 38$) in contrast with conventional risk reduction education with Black adults ($n = 30$) with pre-diabetes. An HbA1C reduction was exhibited in both groups. Mindfulness participants demonstrated reductions in perceived stress, BMI, calorie, carbohydrate and fat intake, and increases in spiritual well-being.

3.4.5.2 Yoga

Based upon a successful pilot (Saper et al. 2009) of a yoga intervention for low back pain in a predominantly minority population, Saper et al. (2013) "conducted a 12-week two-group parallel randomized dosing trial for persons with nonspecific chronic low back pain" in a predominantly minority population ($N = 95$, 80% were nonwhite, 30% had a high school education or less). Both groups demonstrated moderate back pain. Both groups experienced the same yoga protocol with the exception of a once weekly or twice weekly dose. Both groups had statistically significant decreases in pain from baseline to 12 weeks, no difference in outcomes between the two groups. Based on these outcomes, the researchers suggest that a 6-week, once weekly, intervention with strong support for home practice may be effective for long-term benefits.

Johnson et al. (2014) conducted a feasibility study of an internet-based, African dance-modified yoga program for Black women at risk for metabolic syndrome. Johnson—with the assistance of African American experts in teaching yoga in West Africa, West African dance choreography, and an experienced African American physical trainer—designed an intervention culturally congruent with the study target population. The intervention was offered through an internet platform using digital videos. The 4-week yogic dance intervention was delivered daily through video-based instructions located on the study web site. Two themes emerged from the qualitative data: (1) culture is an important aspect of yogic dance and (2) increased social support would enhance yogic dance participation. Participants appreciated an intervention in tune with their own cultural experience. They expressed a preference for connection with the other study participants.

Middleton et al. (2018) (a racially diverse interdisciplinary research team) conducted a feasibility trial of 8 weeks of yoga, adapted for Rheumatoid Arthritis (RA), as a self-care intervention for minorities. Enrolled participants were predominantly Spanish speaking females diagnosed with RA. Twelve of 18 (67%) completed the yoga intervention, all of whom continued to practice yoga 3 months after the end of the study. The researchers concluded that study findings demonstrate the feasibility of offering yoga to a racially/ethnically diverse population with arthritis.

Using a wait-list control, Taylor et al. (2018) conducted a pilot study of an 8-week restorative yoga class with Black breast cancer survivors ($N = 33$). Depression scores at follow-up were significantly lower in the yoga group ($M = 4.78$, SD = 3.56) compared to the control group ($M = 6.91$, SD = 5.86). The researchers conclude that yoga has a beneficial effect on Black breast cancer survivors and warrants further investigation.

Research on CAIH utilization may be biased by not sufficiently sampling minority populations, by not asking the right questions, and by not seeking further understanding from other sources. Qualitative studies with focus groups is one approach to gaining understanding. Another way is to look for historical evidence. Evans (2016) in a content analysis of Black women's memoirs found strong historical evidence of yoga as an approach used by Black women for health and well-being. Given the benefits of yoga for anxiety and depressive conditions, Evans recommends "a greater research focus on yoga as a preventative and corrective intervention" for Black women.

Keosaian et al. (2015) conducted a qualitative study with 19 low-income minority adults (the majority were female, Black, employed, and had public health insurance) participating in a 12-week yoga dosing trial for low back pain. Reported benefits from yoga included decreased back pain, self-efficacy in pain management, mood improvement, and a greater mind-body connection. Identified facilitators to practice included positive relationships with yoga teachers and classmates; barriers included time constraints, lack of motivation, and initial fear of injury.

Kinser and Masho (2015) conducted a qualitative study with pregnant African American teenagers to determine how to create supportive interventions for addressing the stress they experience. Participants reported being primarily interested in yoga, which they perceived as helpful for stress reduction, for combating feelings of isolation, and for some physical aspects of pregnancy. Participants offered suggestions for introducing yoga including ethnically diverse advertising, making classes accessible, encouraging relationship building, and including teaching about managing difficult emotions. The researchers emphasized the importance of designing interventions that meet the needs and desires of the population.

A qualitative study examining perceptions of yoga practice in ethnic minority and low-income adults ($N = 24$; 4 Asian, 5 Black, 6 White)—preliminary to designing an intervention study of yoga for promoting healthy sleep in adults—identified barriers and facilitators to practice (Spadola et al. 2017). Perceptions that "yoga lacks physicality and weight loss benefits, fear of injury, lack of ability/self-efficacy to perform the practices, preference for other physical activities, and scheduling difficulties" act as barriers to considering practice. Facilitators for practice included the importance of qualified engaging yoga instructors, individualized instruction, beginner classes, and encouraging promotional material highlighting the benefits of yoga.

3.5   CAIH for Promoting Health in Vulnerable Populations

Integrative medicine is the clinical practice of integrative health. Integrative medicine provides an ideal fit with disease prevention and health promotion (Oberg et al. 2015). Preventive medicine with its focus on primary, secondary, and tertiary prevention is enhanced by an integrative medicine approach (Li and Katz 2015). At the primary prevention level, CAIH approaches include lifestyle counseling, dietary guidance, stress mitigation techniques, interventions to improve sleep quality, and use of natural products for health promotion. Stress management and lifestyle CAIH innervations act at the secondary prevention level for early intervention and potential reversal with newly diagnosed health problems (e.g., metabolic syndrome). Tertiary prevention employs CAIH interventions for "pain management, symptom control, stress relief, disease management, and risk reduction" for complications.

Saper (2016) suggests solutions for making CAIH more accessible to vulnerable and underserved populations: (1) incorporate services into federally qualified community health centers; (2) make programs available through community-based organizations (e.g., churches, mosques, libraries, community centers, gyms, and veterans centers); (3) develop innovative online tools for improving access (e.g., smartphone apps for stress reduction and monitoring physical activity); (4) make service affordable through lobbying efforts (e.g., insurance reimbursement for CAIH, group visits, and lifestyle modification programs); (5) move to panel-based compensation rather than fee-for-service which will incentivize health and wellness promotion primary and disease treatment secondary; and (6) employ research and quality improvement initiatives to measure and demonstrate the value of CAIH for reduction in health disparities, high patient satisfaction, and lowered costs.

Without the lens of social justice and health equity, CAIH would continue to be available only to the privileged few. Integrative health visionaries see the potential for supporting health in the vulnerable and underserved. An organization called IM4US (Integrative Medicine for the Underserved)—initiated by physicians interested in making CAIH an aware, available, accessible, and affordable option for the underserved—is comprised of "a collaborative, multidisciplinary group of people committed to affordable, accessible integrative healthcare for all, [who] through outreach, education, research, and advocacy, … support those dedicated to promoting health in underserved populations" (Hart 2019, p. 219). Abercrombe (2017), a nurse and past board president, asserts that integrative medicine can contribute to reduced health disparities through enhancing resilience and employing CAIH modalities for stress reduction (e.g., massage). For chronic diseases like diabetes, CAIH employs strategies for lowering blood glucose, reducing inflammation, and prevention of associated conditions (e.g., cardiovascular disease). Through outreach, publications, conferences, and online resources, IM4US offers support to practitioners and the public interested in promoting CAIH for the underserved.

3.6   Nursing's Role

Kinser et al. (2015) describe the ease and relevance of CAIH, in particular self-administered mind-body practices (MBP) for reducing health disparities. Self-administered MBP center on the patient, empowering them to engage actively in their own health. This includes yoga and meditation. Nurses are in an ideal position to facilitate CAIH access through role modeling and teaching MBP for the vulnerable and underserved. Nurses can

- Gain first-hand experiences with a variety of CAIH modalities through incorporating them in self-care practice.
- Become knowledgeable about CAIH and the underserved by joining organizations and attending conferences (IM4US, American Holistic Nursing Association, International Integrative Nursing Symposium).
- Acquire knowledge, skills, and certification in CAIH modalities. Advanced practice nurses can complete integrative health fellowships for advanced certification.
- Design and conduct research.
- Serve on boards associated with improving health.
- Create programs for the vulnerable and underserved (Rancour & Haley 2017).
- Advocate for the integration of efficacious CAIH modalities for primary prevention.

3.7   Summary and Conclusions/Final Words

At its greatest vision an integrative health perspective calls for a major change of philosophy about what constitutes health and the role of individuals, organizations, healthcare providers, and the infrastructure in improving the health of the vulnerable and underserved. In the meantime, much progress has been made to bring awareness of the value and necessity of access to CAIH approaches.

References

Abercrombe P (2017) Integrative medicine is the key to reducing health disparities. *Massage Magazine*. https://www.massagemag.com/integrative-medicine-reducing-health-disparities-87632/

Bailey ZD, Krieger N, Agénor M, Graves J, Linos N, Bassett MT (2017) Structural racism and health inequities in the USA: evidence and interventions. Lancet 389(10077):1453–1463

Bains SS, Egede LE (2011) Association of health literacy with complementary and alternative medicine use: a cross-sectional study in adult primary care patients. BMC Complement Altern Med 11(1):138

Barnett MC, Cotroneo M, Purnell J, Martin D, Mackenzie E, Fishman A (2003) Use of CAM in local African-American communities: community-partnered research. J Natl Med Assoc 95(10):943–950

Bazargan M, Ani CO, Hindman DW, Bazargan-Hejazi S, Baker RS, Bell D, Rodriquez M (2008) Correlates of complementary and alternative medicine utilization in depressed, underserved African American and Hispanic patients in primary care settings. J Altern Complement Med 14(5):537–544

Berg J, Morphew T, Tran J, Kilgore D, Galant SP (2016) Prevalence of complementary and alternative medicine usage in Vietnamese American asthmatic children. Clin Pediatr 55(2):157–164

Bishop FL, Lewith GT (2010) Who uses CAM? A narrative review of demographic characteristics and health factors associated with CAM use. eCAM 7(1):11–28

Brown CM, Barner JC, Richards KM, Bohman T (2007) Patterns of complementary and alternative medicine use in African Americans. J Altern Complement Med 13(7):751–758

Burke A, Nahin RL, Stussman BJ (2015) Limited health knowledge as a reason for non-use of four common complementary health practices. PLoS One 10(6):e0129336

Chao MT, Handley MA, Quan J, Sarka U, Ratanawongsa N, Schillinger D (2015) Disclosure of complementary health approaches among low income and racially diverse safety net patients with diabetes. Patient Educ Couns 98:1360–1366

Charlson ME, Loizzo J, Moadel A, Neale M, Newman C, Olivo E, Wolf E, Peterson JC (2014) Contemplative self-healing in women breast cancer survivors: a pilot study in underserved minority women shows improvement in quality of life and reduced stress. BMC Complement Altern Med 14(1):349

Clarke TC, Black LI, Stussman BJ, Barnes PM, Nahin RL (2015) Trends in the use of complementary health approaches among adults: United States, 2002–2012. Natl Health Stat Rep (79):1–16

Clarke TC, Barnes PM, Black LI, Stussman BJ, Nahin RL (2018) Use of yoga, meditation, and chiropractors among US adults aged 18 and over. US Department of Health and Human Services, Centers for Disease Control and Prevention, National Center for Health Statistics

Coughlin SS, Yoo W, Whitehead MS, Smith SA (2015) Advancing breast cancer survivorship among African-American women. Breast Cancer Res Treat 153(2):253–261

di Sarsina PR, Alivia M, Guadagni P (2012) Traditional, complementary and alternative medical systems and their contribution to personalisation, prediction and prevention in medicine—person-centred medicine. EPMA J 3(1):15

Dresner D, Gergen Barnett K, Resnick K, Laird LD, Gardiner P (2016) Listening to their words: a qualitative analysis of integrative medicine group visits in an urban underserved medical setting. Pain Med 17(6):1183–1191

Evans S (2016) Yoga in 42 African American women's memoirs reveal hidden tradition of health. Int J Yoga 9(1):85

Green RR, Santoro N, Allshouse AA, Neal-Perry G, Derby C (2017) Prevalence of complementary and alternative medicine and herbal remedy use in Hispanic and non-Hispanic white women: results from the study of women's health across the nation. J Altern Complement Med 23(10):805–811

Hart J (2019) IM4US: integrative medicine for the underserved. Altern Complement Ther 25(4):219–221

Ho DB, Nguyen J, Liu MA, Nguyen AL, Kilgore DB (2015) Use of and interests in complementary and alternative medicine by Hispanic patients of a community health center. J Am Board Fam Med 2015(28):175–183

Institute of Medicine. Committee on the Use of Complementary Alternative Medicine the American Public (2005) Complementary and alternative medicine in the United States. National Academies Press, Washington, DC

Johnson CC, Taylor AG, Anderson JG, Jones RA, Whaley DE (2014) Feasibility and acceptability of an internet-based, African dance-modified yoga program for African American women with or at risk for metabolic syndrome. J Yoga Phys Ther 4:174

Jones D, Cohen L, Rieber AG, Urbauer D, Fellman B, Fisch MJ, Nazario A (2018) Complementary and alternative medicine use in minority and medically underserved oncology patients: assessment and implications. Integrative cancer therapies. 17(2):371–379

Keosaian JE, Lemaster CM, Dresner D, Godersky ME, Paris R, Sherman KJ, Saper RB (2015) "We're all in this together": a qualitative study of predominantly low-income minority participants in a yoga trial for chronic low back pain. Complement Ther Med 24:34–39

Kinser P, Masho S (2015) "I just start crying for no reason": the experience of stress and depression in pregnant, urban, African-American adolescents and their perception of yoga as a management strategy. Womens Health Issues 25(2):142–148

Kinser PA, Robins JLW, Masho SW (2015) Self-administered mind-body practices for reducing health disparities: An interprofessional opinion and call to action. Evidence-Based Complementary and Alternative Medicine 2016:6 pages.

Lindberg NM, Vega-López S, Arias-Gastelum M, Stevens VJ (2019) Alternative medicine methods used for weight loss and diabetes control by overweight and obese Hispanic immigrant women. Hisp Health Care Int 18(2):49–54

Li A, Katz DL (2015) Disease prevention and health promotion: how integrative medicine fits. Am J Prev Med 49(5):S230–S240

Lyons T, Womack VY, Cantrell WD, Kenemore T (2019) Mindfulness-based relapse prevention in a jail drug treatment program. Subst Use Misuse 54(1):57–64

Middleton KR, Ward MM, Moonaz SH, López MM, Tataw-Ayuketah G, Yang L, Acevedo AT, Brandon Z, Wallen GR (2018) Feasibility and assessment of outcome measures for yoga as self-care for minorities with arthritis: a pilot study. Pilot Feasibility Stud 4(53):1–11

Nguyen H, Sorkin DDH, Billimek DJ, Kaplan DSH, Greenfield DS, Ngo-Metzger DQ (2014) Complementary and alternative medicine (CAM) use among non-Hispanic white, Mexican American, and Vietnamese American patients with type 2 diabetes. J Health Care Poor Underserved 25(4):1941

Oberg E, Guarneri M, Herman P, Walsh T, Wostrel A (2015) Integrative health and medicine: today's answer to affordable healthcare. In: Integrative healthcare policy consortium, pp 1–16

Pinzon-Perez H (ed) (2016) Complementary, alternative, and integrative health: a multicultural perspective. Wiley, Hoboken, NJ

Rancour P, Haley L (2017) The stone soup project: a model for the delivery of holistic health services to under-served populations in the community. Altern Complement Ther 23(5):171–175

Rhee TG, Evans RL, McAlpine DD, Johnson PJ (2016) Racial/ethnic differences in the use of complementary and alternative medicine in us adults with moderate mental distress: results from the 2012 National Health Interview Survey. J Prim Care Community Health 8(2):43–54

Robles B, Upchurch DM, Kuo T (2017) Comparing complementary and alternative medicine use with or without including prayer as a modality in a local and diverse United States jurisdiction. Front Public Health 5:56

Rush CL, Lobo T, Serrano A, Blasini M, Campos C, Graves KD (2016) Complementary and alternative medicine use and Latina breast cancer survivors' symptoms and functioning. Healthcare 4(80):1–14.

Saper RB (2016) Integrative medicine and health disparities. Glob Adv Health Med 5(1):5–8. https://doi.org/10.7453/gahmj.2015.133

Saper RB, Sherman KJ, Cullum-Dugan D, Davis RB, Phillips RS, Culpepper L (2009) Yoga for chronic low back pain in a predominantly minority population: a pilot randomized controlled trial. Altern Ther Health Med 15(6):18

Saper RB, Boah AR, Keosaian J, Cerrada C, Weinberg J, Sherman KJ (2013) Comparing once-versus twice-weekly yoga classes for chronic low back pain in predominantly low-income minorities: a randomized dosing trial. Evid Based Complement Alternat Med 2013:658030

Shelley BM, Sussman AL, Williams RL, Segal AR, Crabtree BF (2009) 'They don't ask me so I don't tell them': patient-clinician communication about traditional, complementary, and alternative medicine. Ann Fam Med 7(2):139–147

Spadola CE, Rottapel R, Khandpur N, Kontos E, Bertisch SM, Johnson DA, Quante M, Khalsa SBS, Saper RB, Redline S (2017) Enhancing yoga participation: a qualitative investigation of barriers and facilitators to yoga among predominantly racial/ethnic minority, low-income adults. Complement Ther Clin Pract 29:97–104

Taylor TR, Barrow J, Makambi K, Sheppard V, Wallington SF, Martin C, Greene D, Yeruva S, Horton S (2018) A restorative yoga intervention for African-American breast cancer survivors: a pilot study. J Racial Ethn Health Disparities 5(1):62–72

Wahbeh H, Elsas SM, Oken BS (2008) Mind-body interventions: applications in neurology. Neurology 70(24):2321–2328

Ward J, Humphries K, Webb C, Ramcharan M (2013) Review of the use of complementary and alternative medicine by non-Hispanic blacks. Topics Integr Health Care 4:1

Witt C (2017) A new definition of integrative health. Institute for Integrative Health. https://tiih.org/who/blog/new-definition-integrative-health/

Woods-Giscombe CL, Gaylord SA, Li Y, Brintz CE, Bangdiwala SI, Buse JB, Leniek K (2019) A mixed-methods, randomized clinical trial to examine feasibility of a mindfulness-based stress management and diabetes risk reduction intervention for African Americans with prediabetes. Evid Based Complement Alternat Med 2019:3962623

Mindfulness and Stress Reduction Strategies with Undergraduate and Graduate Nursing Students

4

Amber Vermeesch and Patricia Cox

4.1 Introduction

Nursing students face higher and different levels of perceived stress with adverse health outcomes compared to other students. Literature has linked perceived stress to reduced physical/psychological health including depression, increased sickness/absence, increased staff turnover, and poor job and academic performance. Nursing educators must provide coping strategies to nursing students at all levels, to enable them to attain unique skill sets to build resiliency and reduce perceived stress while managing physical and mental stressors of challenging nursing curricula. This chapter will explore integrative health nursing strategies to reduce perceived stress among undergraduate and graduate nursing students.

4.2 Background

4.2.1 Perceived Stress Among Undergraduate and Graduate Nursing Students

Perceived stress is defined by Lazarus (1966) as the perception that external demands are beyond the perceived ability of an individual to cope. Small and large stressors may be a daily occurrence for many of us; however, feeling overwhelmed is a common experience of undergraduate and graduate nursing students. An American Psychological Association (APA) (2010) survey found that perceived stress not only affects physical and emotional health but also disrupts families. Some factors associated with perceived stress unique to nursing and other medical disciplines that provide intimate patient care include Inappropriate Patient Sexual Behavior (IPSB).

A. Vermeesch (✉) · P. Cox
School of Nursing, University of Portland, Portland, OR, USA
e-mail: vermeesc@up.edu; coxp@up.edu

© Springer Nature Switzerland AG 2021
A. Vermeesch (ed.), *Integrative Health Nursing Interventions for Vulnerable Populations*, https://doi.org/10.1007/978-3-030-60043-3_4

In nursing, IPSB is defined as "verbal or physical act of an explicit, or perceived sexual nature which is unacceptable within the social context in which it is carried out" (Johnson et al. 2006; Wyss and Vermeesch 2019). Nurses who have been working for many years may have developed coping mechanisms to handle stressful work environments, nursing students may be unable to navigate such patient situations while also learning the art and science of nursing (Wyss and Vermeesch 2019). In addition, nursing and other professions involved with patient care, experience the emotional toll of death and ethical dilemmas on caregivers (Keogh 2019; Rainer et al. 2018). These factors have a cumulative effect on undergraduate and graduate nursing students and university health centers are reporting a dramatic increase in the number of students reporting anxiety and depression (Greeson et al. 2014). The mental health challenges reported include difficulties with personal relationships, campus engagement, and graduation rates. These numbers are sharply rising during the current COVID-19 pandemic (Conrad et al. 2020; Rajkumar 2020).

4.3 Nursing Stressors

4.3.1 Undergraduate Nursing Stressors

Nursing students must meet rigorous academic standards and the demands of a complex healthcare environment. Undergraduate stressors include time management, academic obligations and performance, clinical rotations, overall mental and physical health, social and family life, finances, NCLEX, and finding a job after graduation (Barber et al. 2018). It is well known that perceived stress is a major factor in nursing school and increases as students' progress through their program (Brown et al. 2016). Stressors of undergraduate and graduate nursing school can have a negative impact and effect on a student's well-being, academic success, and future career development (Garcia-Williams et al. 2014).

4.3.2 Graduate Nursing Stressors

Graduate nursing students are particularly vulnerable to stress due to the multiple demands of school, work, family obligations, financial worries, and performance in clinical rotations (Brown et al. 2016; Enns et al. 2018). Baldwin (2013) reported in her research with doctoral nursing students in the United Kingdom, that students had multiple challenges with family and social commitments. She identified similar challenges to Barber et al. (2018) that included: balancing time, work, personal life, and academic responsibilities. According to Bond et al. (2013) increased perceived stress decreases medical student's ability to connect with patients. Communicating and connecting with patients is key to the role of nurses and decreasing perceived stress then would be paramount to engage patients and optimize health and wellness. Connection between caregiver and patient ties into two principles of integrative nursing through the idea that integrative nursing is person-centered and relationship-based and focuses on the health and wellbeing of caregivers as well as those they serve (Kreitzer and Koithan 2014).

4.4 Integrative Interventions Strategies to Reduce Perceived Stress in Nursing Students

Effective and sustainable interventions to reduce students' perceived stress should be integrative and think of students as whole persons—mind, body, and spirit. Additionally, they should include complementary approaches to optimizing wellness and as such, have the capacity to reduce potentially negative health effects and prepare students to manage their future stress (Stillwell et al. 2017).

A body of literature now supports mindfulness having a positive effect on both physical and mental health (Felton et al. 2015). Mindfulness mediation may improve coping skills that enhances cognitive functioning, reduces perceived stress and improves disposition in students (Spadaro and Hunker 2016). In 2017, Alsaraireh and Aloush compared the effectiveness of mindfulness meditation versus physical exercise in managing depression in nursing students. In this study, 181 nursing students participated and were randomly assigned to either physical exercise ($n = 90$) or mindfulness meditation ($n = 91$). Pre- and post-intervention students completed The Center for Epidemiologic Studies Depression Scale. Alsaraireh and Aloush found both therapies were effective in the treatment of depressive symptoms. Mindfulness meditation, however, was more effective than the physical exercise.

Recently, Spadaro and Hunker (2016) explored the effect of an online mindfulness meditation program on stress, mood, and cognition in nursing students enrolled in both undergraduate and graduate nursing programs at a mid-Atlantic university. The students were provided with the mindfulness intervention in an asynchronous online format over 8 weeks with a 16-week follow-up. They used the Perceived Stress Scale (PSS), Hospital Anxiety and Depression Scale (HADS), and Attention Network Test (ANT) to measure outcomes. The authors found a significant decrease in stress and a decreasing trend in anxiety for those that practiced mindfulness meditation daily to weekly. Concentration, and attention accuracy improved. Mindfulness stress reduction programs are helpful even if delivered in a distant learning format.

Mindfulness has been used to overcome the multiple challenges of ethnic minority students in an undergraduate nursing program (Young-Brice and Dreifuerst 2019). Positive associations of mindfulness (e.g., acknowledging the ability to have awareness of thoughts, feelings, and ability to adapt to college) and negative consequences with lower levels of mindfulness were revealed in a qualitative study with 20 undergraduate nursing students. The authors concluded that using consistent mindfulness techniques could positively influence coping skills for college stressors resulting in overall student success and retention of ethnic minority and first-generation students in a nursing program (Young-Brice and Dreifuerst 2019).

To support graduate nursing students in reducing perceived stress, a nursing school in the Pacific Northwest developed an evidence-based mindfulness meditation focused intervention. Results of this year-long effort demonstrated a trend in reduction of PSS scores between the data time points. Of the students surveyed, 58.4% reported the experience helped manage their stress (e.g., improved very much/vastly improved) and 58.3% reported daily/weekly frequency of practice. As expected, there was a positive correlation between hours worked and increased stress. Additionally, a positive correlation surfaced between daily practice and reduction in perceived stress with the total score on the Perceived Stress Scale T1 M = 21 and T4 M = 15.75. The authors conclusion was that developing a self-care routine of mindfulness meditation may assist graduate students in reduction of perceived stress (Cox et al. 2019).

To address identified stressors among undergraduate nursing students including transitioning into the academic environment, rigorous courses and clinicals, a nursing school in the Pacific Northwest developed an evidence-based peer mentor program, especially to increase retention of minority populations and high financial need students. Retention and financial need have been cited by other authors as stressors for minority and first-generation students (Barber et al. 2018; Brown et al. 2016; Garcia-Williams et al. 2014; Young-Brice and Dreifuerst 2019). This program is known as BUDDY-UP and freshman met with peer mentors of similar backgrounds (e.g., ethnically diverse, male, and first-generation students). Evaluation of BUDDY-UP included quantitative and qualitative data; findings inform future peer mentoring best practices and support sustainability in traditional BSN programs. While perceived stress was not specifically measured, qualitative findings revealed, "He helped me… gave me tips on how he manages time and manages difficult moments." Also, "It was so nice to meet someone who had gone through the coursework and survived it, it gave me confidence for success." The first year of this program increased retention from 86% to 92% (Majors 2017).

4.5   Interventions to Reduce Perceived Stress in Other Disciplines

A meta-analysis conducted by Yusufov et al. (2019) evaluated the efficacy of stress reduction interventions used for undergraduate and graduate students. Type of students were not delineated. Results indicated that most of the interventions were effective in decreasing perceived stress in students. Cognitive interventions such as therapies to affect coping skills, social support, and included behavioral therapy were more effective in reducing perceived stress. Participants in both the long- and short-term interventions showed significant reductions in perceived stress relative to control groups. Tailoring interventions toward a specific group and outcome proved more effective in reducing stress-related outcomes.

Being present in the moment is a strategy that has decreased stress, improved mood and academic performance in college students (Greeson et al. 2014). There are multiple studies that have demonstrated the effectiveness of mindfulness interventions on perceived stress levels of undergraduate and graduate students. One unique program is Mindfulness Based Stress Reduction (MBSR) developed by Jon Kabat-Zinn. It uses a structured program of meditation with yoga that focuses on the present to allow awareness of, and use of one's innate abilities to manage pain, stress, and illness (Kabat-Zinn and Hanh 2013; Plummer et al. 2018). Greeson et al. (2014) demonstrated that their specialized Koru, mindfulness program was effective in reducing stress, improving well-being, and prompting sleep in undergraduate and graduate students. Their program included mindfulness, meditation, and mind-body skills which is similar to MBSR and other mindfulness program already mentioned.

Psychology students have similar stressors to graduate nursing students; most notable is in developing specific skill sets to provide therapeutic and clinic services to others (Myers et al. 2012). Beck and Verticchio (2014) reported the results of a mindfulness practice on counseling skills of graduate students who were communication science and disorders majors. The mindfulness practice included 5 min of stretching, seated breathing, and 2 min of reflective writing. They found that counseling confidence increased and scores on the Perceived Stress Scale (PSS) decreased. The students were aware of being more mindful in their counseling as well as their expressed overall well-being.

O'Neill et al. (2019) investigated the relationship between self-care and academic stress in social work students. To improve the practice of self-care for academic success and career longevity, they surveyed 90 social work students at the bachelors and master's level. Those that practiced self-care had lower levels of perceived stress. As students progressed through the program, they had less perceived stress despite the type of self-care practiced. They concluded that social work programs need to teach self-care and encourage practice.

Others have used their own developed mindfulness programs to manage perceived stress. Swift et al. (2017) set out to test the effectiveness of mindfulness training for psychotherapist students. The randomized-controlled crossover trial included 40 graduate student psychotherapists from two universities. They were either assigned to the mindfulness group or control group. The mindfulness group received a 5-week mindfulness training program while those in the control group received the program only after a 5-week no-contact period. The mindfulness training group showed significantly greater improvements in being mindful and had higher levels of being present during treatment sessions over the control group. No differences were seen between the two groups by clients in their session ratings or effectiveness. The study did have a clear benefit for the well-being of students and satisfaction similar to other studies (Felton et al. 2015). Consequently, other disciplines may want to provide mindfulness in their curricula as part of the practicum training experience. Other formats in mindfulness training may be more effective than the one used in this study.

In addition, Dye et al. (2020) found that graduate counseling students benefitted from mindfulness training at the beginning and end of each class over 13 weeks. The training included a combination of meditation, muscle relaxation, yoga, mindful walking and exercises followed by reflective discussions. The students reported enhanced relaxation, increased awareness for self-care, and better connection between mindfulness and overall well-being. The mindfulness training aided the students in developing self-care strategies and thereby gaining the additional tools they might need to help their clients. The authors concluded that incorporating mindfulness in a weekly or daily counseling classes was both feasible and beneficial for promoting relaxation and self-care.

4.6 Conclusion and Next Steps

The authors conclude that the delivery platform of mindfulness does not matter in terms of effectiveness. What does matter is consistent technique influences coping of nursing students, particularly of ethnically diverse students, in building resilience. In order to reduce perceived stress in undergraduate and graduate nursing students, faculty would be wise to include strategies for self-care and encourage students to participate. Faculty should be trained to assess stress in graduate and undergraduate nursing students. In addition, faculty should be prepared to refer students to appropriate mental health services. As discovered by White et al. (2019), curriculum-based mindfulness strategies must be integrated throughout all courses to ensure widespread dissemination. Integration of mindfulness practices into a graduate nursing curriculum may decrease stress and improve health outcomes (Plummer et al. 2018). Research to explore stress levels in educational programs can assist educators in designing and introducing stress reduction strategies and introduce interventions to decrease the deleterious effects of stress (Brown et al. 2016).

References

Alsaraireh FA, Aloush SM (2017) Mindfulness meditation versus physical exercise in the management of depression among nursing students. J Nurs Educ 56(10):599–604

American Psychological Association (2010) APA survey raises concern about health impact of stress on children and families. https://www.apa.org/news/press/releases/2010/11/stress-in-america.aspx

Baldwin S (2013) Exploring the experiences of nurses studying professional doctorates. Br J Nurs 2298:476–478. https://doi.org/10.12968/bjon.2013.22.8.476

Barber H, Vermeesch A, Fenner S, McDonagh L (2018) Road less traveled: stressors & coping strategies of undergraduate nursing students. In: Poster presentation at Western Institute of Nursing's 51th Annual Communication Nursing Research Conferences, Spokane, WA, April 11–14, 2018

Beck AR, Verticchio H (Fall, 2014) Counseling and mindfulness practice with graduate students in communication sciences and disorders. Contemp Issues Commun Sci Disord 41:133–148

Bond AR, Mason HF, Lemaster CM, Shaw SE, Mullin CS, Holick EA, Saper RB (April 2013) Embodied health: the effects of mind-body course for medical students. Med Educ Online 18:1–8. https://doi.org/10.3402/meo.v18i0.20699

Brown K, Anderson-Johnson P, McPherson AN (2016) Academic-related stress among graduate students in nursing in a Jamaican school of nursing. Nurse Educ Pract 20:117–124

Conrad R, Rayala H, Menon M, Vora K (2020) Universities' response to supporting mental health of college students during the COVID-19 pandemic. *Psychiatric Times*

Cox P, Potter P, Vermeesch A, Stillwell S (2019) Effect of mindfulness on perceived stress by graduate nursing students. In: Podium Presentation at 3rd International Integrative Nursing Symposium, Galway, Ireland, May 22–24, 2019

Dye L, Burke MG, Wolf C (2020) Teaching mindfulness for the self-care and well-being of counselors-in-training. J Creat Ment Health 15(2):140–153. https://doi.org/10.1080/1540138 3.2019.1642171

Enns A, Eldridge GD, Montgomery C, Gonzalez VM (2018) Perceived stress, coping strategies, and emotional intelligence: a cross sectional study of university students in helping disciplines. Nurse Educ Today 68:226–231

Felton TM, Coates L, Christopher JC (2015) Impact of mindfulness training on counseling students' perceptions of stress. Mindfulness 6:159–169. https://doi.org/10.1007/s12671-013-0240-8

Garcia-Williams AG, Moffitt L, Kaslow NJ (2014) Mental health and suicidal behavior among graduate students. Acad Psychiatry 38:554–560. https://doi.org/10.1007/s40596-014-0041-y

Greeson JM, Juberg MK, Maytan M, James K, Rogers H (2014) A randomized controlled trial of koru: a mindfulness program for college students and other emerging adults. J Am Coll Health 62(4):222–233

Johnson C, Knight C, Alderman N (2006) Challenges associated with the definition and assessment of inappropriate sexual behaviour amongst individuals with an acquired neurological impairment. Brain Inj 20:687–693

Kabat-Zinn J, Hanh TN (2013) Full catastrophe living (revised edition): using the wisdom of your body and mind to face stress, pain, and illness. Bantam Books, New York

Keogh K (2019) Finding time to talk through the emotional toll of caring [Editorial]. Cancer Nursing Practice 18(5):5. https://doi.org/10.7748/cnp.18.5.5.s1

Kreitzer MJ, Koithan M (eds) (2014) Integrative nursing. Oxford Press, New York

Lazarus RS (1966) Psychological stress and the coping process. McGraw-Hill, New York

Majors E (2017) BUDDY-UP: an educational innovation enhancing student nurse retention. In: Poster Presentation at American Association of Colleges of Nursing's 2017 baccalaureate education conference, Atlanta, GA, November 16–18, 2017

Myers SB, Sweeney AC, Popick V, Wesley K, Bordfeld A, Fingerhut R (2012) Self-care and perceived stress levels among psychology graduate students. Training Educ Profess Psychol 6(1):55–66. https://doi.org/10.1037/a0026534

O'Neill M, Slater GY, Batt D (2019) Social work student self-care and academic stress. J Soc Work Educ 55(1):141–152. https://doi.org/10.1080/10437797.2018.1491359

Plummer C, Cloyd E, Doersam JK, Dietrich MS, Hande KA (2018) Mindfulness in a graduate nursing curriculum: a randomized controlled study. Holist Nurs Pract 32(4):189–195

Rainer J, Schneider JK, Lorenz RA (2018) Ethical dilemmas in nursing: an integrative review. J Clin Nurs 27(19–20):3446–3461

Rajkumar RP (2020) COVID-19 and mental health: a review of the existing literature. Asian J Psychiatr 52:102066. Advance online publication. https://doi.org/10.1016/j.ajp.2020.102066

Spadaro KC, Hunker DF (2016) Exploring the effects of an online asynchronous mindfulness meditation intervention with nursing students on stress, mood, and cognition: a descriptive study. Nurse Educ Today 39:163–169

Stillwell SB, Vermeesch AL, Scott JG (2017) Interventions to reduce perceived stress among graduate students: a systematic review with implications for evidenced-based practice. Worldviews Evid Based Nurs 14(6):507–513

Swift JK, Callahan JL, Dunn R, Brecht K, Ivanovic M (2017) A randomized-controlled crossover trial of mindfulness for student psychotherapists. Training Educ Profess Psychol 11(4):235–242. https://doi.org/10.1037/tep0000154

White MA, Whittaker SD, Gores AM, Allswede D (2019) Evaluation of a self-care intervention to improve student mental health administered through a distance-learning course. Am J Health Sci 50(4):213–224. https://doi.org/10.1080/19325037.2019.1616012

Wyss H, Vermeesch A (2019) Inappropriate patient sexual behavior in nursing education. Arch Women Health Care 2(1):1–1

Young-Brice A, Dreifuerst KT (2019) Exploration of mindfulness among ethnic minority undergraduate nursing students. Nurse Educ 44(6):316–320. https://doi.org/10.1097/NNE.0000000000000629

Yusufov M, Nicoloro-SantaBarbara J, Grey NE, Moyer A, Lobel M (2019) Meta-analytic evaluation of stress reduction interventions for undergraduate and graduate students. Int J Stress Manag 26(2):132–145

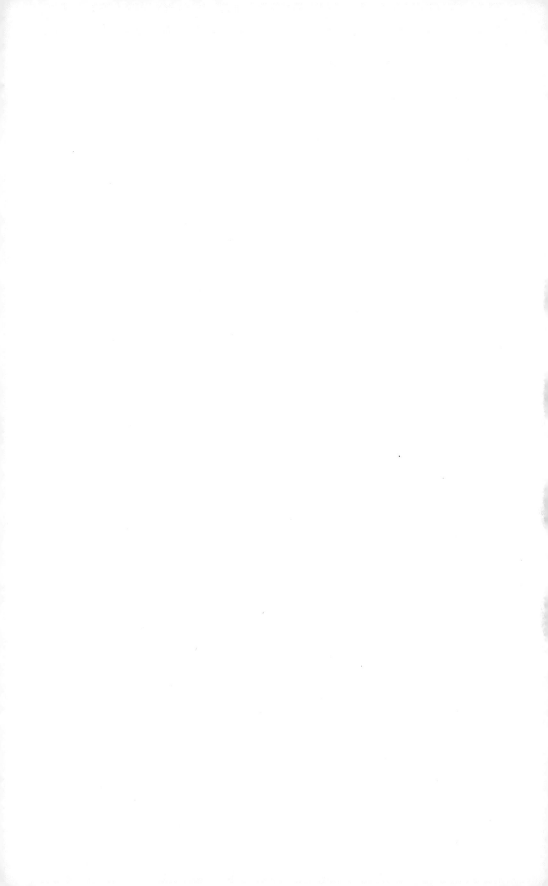

Caring for Ourselves as Nurses

5

Cynthia Backer and Judith Ulibarri

When we change the conversation, we change the future.
Juanita Brown

5.1 Introduction

Do any of these situations sound familiar to you?
Have you ever felt like you could never work hard enough?
Do you experience back pain, migraines, aches, depression, and/or high blood pressure?
Do you not answer your phone or avoid social events in your personal life?
Do you commit to projects that you should probably say no to?

If any of these situations apply to you or other nurses, *know you are not alone.* Currently many nurses are less healthy than the average American and are more likely to be overweight, have higher levels of stress and get less sleep (ANA 2016). Sixty-eight percent of nurses reported putting the health, safety, and wellness of their patients before their own (ANA 2020).

In addition to being a nurse, you may also be in a caregiving role in your personal life; perhaps you are taking care of children, a parent, or an ill friend. You may have experienced worry, loneliness, or difficulty sleeping, all potential signs and symptoms of caregiving/compassion fatigue. What is important to know is caregiving/compassion fatigue is not a weakness; it is a sign of being human (Germer and Neff 2019).

C. Backer (✉)
Home Health, PeaceHealth System, Vancouver, WA, USA
e-mail: cbacker@peacehealth.org

J. Ulibarri
Integrative Health and Wellness, VA Portland Health Care Systems, Portland, OR, USA
e-mail: Judith.ulibarri@va.gov

© Springer Nature Switzerland AG 2021
A. Vermeesch (ed.), *Integrative Health Nursing Interventions for Vulnerable Populations*, https://doi.org/10.1007/978-3-030-60043-3_5

If any of these situations are resonating with you, how can you care for yourself? You did not intentionally drop your needs to the bottom of your priorities. You most likely acknowledge self-care is essential to be healthy, to be a role model and to continue to provide best care. You can probably recall sometimes during your life when you experienced balance and self-care. But other times you most likely spent more time giving to others than caring for yourself. It is easy to become depleted, experiencing a deficit in your own well-being. Self-care activities may or may not have been an option, or perhaps they simply were enough to fill yourself back up. You may be depleting at a faster rate than you are giving out.

Why then, is it so hard to be compassionate to ourselves? To use a scenario from the airlines, why are we consistently putting oxygen masks on others before ourselves? Is it possible we are fatigued from being compassionate? We might even know about integrative nursing and how it includes focusing on the health and well-being of caregivers as well as those they serve (Kreitzer and Koithan 2019). It can be challenging to utilize available resources even if we are aware of them. What is stopping us from better balancing ourselves? Let us look at how we as nurses might find ourselves in a place of compassion fatigue.

5.2   Defining Nursing Compassion Fatigue

How could being compassionate cause fatigue for nurses? Dr. Kate Sheppard recently researched this potential situation among registered nurses and shared:

> "Ideally, as nurses, we should feel satisfied with our work and derive satisfaction from providing excellent care. Compassion fatigue has been defined as loss of satisfaction that comes from doing one's job well, or job-related distress that out weighs job satisfaction." (Sheppard 2016)

The idea of nurses experiencing compassion fatigue is not new. Carla Joinson introduced the concept to the nursing community in 1992 in her *Nursing* magazine article. Joinson credited Doris Chase, a crisis counselor, for the term compassion fatigue. Chase states "the elements of burnout can occur in any setting, a unique form of it, compassion fatigue, affects people in caregiving professions…nurses are very susceptible to it." (Joinson 1992).

Nurses' compassion fatigue can be evidenced in many ways (Sheppard 2016). For many nurses, the first symptoms are emotional. Some nurses are more forgetful, have a decreased attention span or are more irritable. Symptoms may progress to physical symptoms such as inability to get a good night's sleep, exhaustion, and physical illnesses. These symptoms can lead to apathy, absenteeism, anger, and even increased use of alcohol and drugs.

Joinson pointed out nurses' personalities can lead them toward compassion fatigue but awareness and response to potential situations are key (1992). She shares three core issues in compassion fatigue for caregivers, such as nurses, identified by Rev. Stephen Wende:

1. Caregivers may perform a number of concrete functions, but the essential product they deliver is themselves. This can be very taxing. They have to renew themselves, building themselves back up, or they are in trouble.
    2. Human need is infinite. Caregivers tend to feel "I can always give a little more," but sometimes they just can't help.
    3. Caregivers fill multiple roles that can be psychologically conflicting…They can lose a lot of energy shifting roles. The trick is to be conscious of each change and ease into it gracefully, without fighting the new role (Joinson 1992).

5.3   Tools to Identify Compassion Fatigue

Various measurement tools have been developed that can help indicate the presence of compassion fatigue in nurses. One of the first scales, the Social Readjustment Rating Scale (SRRS), focused on measuring stress. The SRRS was developed in 1967, by psychiatrists Thomas Holmes and Richard Rahe studying whether stress contributes to illness. They surveyed more than 5000 medical patients and asked them to say whether they had experience in any of a series of 43 life events in the previous 2 years. While this scale can be helpful for some nurses, one of the weaknesses cited has been the scale's lack of allowing for variability in how stress is handled, say for example, due to cultural approaches (MindTools 2020).

A more helpful, specific and beneficial measurement tool in measuring compassion fatigue and compassion satisfaction is the Professional Quality of Life Measure (ProQOL 2020). The ProQOL 5, first developed in 1995, is the most commonly used measure of the negative and positive effects of helping others who experience suffering and trauma. The tool is easy to use, can be given individually or in groups and can be given online (ProQOL Slide Set 2012).

Figure 5.1 shows the sub-scales of the ProQOL for compassion satisfaction, burnout, and compassion fatigue. Here are the definitions related to nurses:

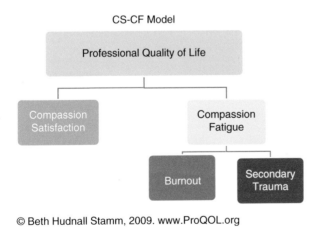

© Beth Hudnall Stamm, 2009. www.ProQOL.org

Fig. 5.1 ProQOL sub-scales of compassion satisfaction, burnout, and compassion fatigue (© Beth Hudnall Stamm 2009)

Compassion Satisfaction - positive aspects of working as a nurse
Compassion Fatigue - negative aspects of working as a nurse
Burnout - worn out due to work; related hopelessness and feelings of inefficacy
Secondary Trauma – occurs less frequently; frightened or traumatized due to exposure to someone else's trauma (ProQOL Slide Set 2012).

More recently, additional tools are available to nurses to assess and reflect on their self-care and resilience, contributing to compassion satisfaction. Two highly recommended tools that have been validated are: (1) Integrative Health and Wellness Assessment (short form)—International Nurse Coach Association (Dossey 2015) and (2) Skovholt Practitioner Professional Resiliency and Self-Care Inventory (2014).

The INCA Integrative Health and Wellness Assessment short form is simple and easy to use. Information can be gathered quickly on life balance/satisfaction, relationships, spiritual, mental, emotional, physical/nutrition, physical/exercise, physical/weight, environment, and health responsibility (Dossey et al. 2015). Also, the Skovholt Practitioner Professional Resiliency and Self-Care Inventory is an easy-to-use method for self-reflection and for use in groups. It covers professional vitality, personal vitality, professional stress, and personal stress (Skovholt and Trotter-Mathison 2016).

5.4 How to Care for Ourselves

In her newly revised book, *Compassion Fatigue and Burnout in Nursing*, Dr. Vidette Todaro-Franceschi shares her ART Model for Enhancing Professional Quality of Life as a healing model for our nursing community:

Acknowledging – acknowledgement of a feeling or problem
Recognizing – explore your options, reexamine your intentions, reaffirm your purpose
Turning – reconnect with yourself and others (p. 66, Todaro-Franceschi 2019)

Let us look at each of these steps individually to prevent or reduce compassion fatigue for each of us as nurses.

5.4.1 Acknowledging

The first step is caring for yourself with ART is noticing how you are feeling in this present moment. This includes allowing all feelings—positive, negative, emotional, and physical. Have compassion for yourself. Notice how you feel, without judgement. Are there any problems or concerns? If a certain situation is bothering you, notice that. For example, you may have personal circumstances impacting you now or be in a challenging work environment.

Francoise Mathieu, in her article *Running on Empty: Compassion Fatigue in Health Professionals* reinforces the need to acknowledge how you are feeling.

"Learning to recognize one's own symptoms of compassion fatigue as a two-fold purpose: firstly, it can serve as an important "check-in" process for a helper who has been feeling unhappy and dissatisfied but did not have the words to explain what was happening to them, and secondly, it can allow them to develop a warning system for themselves." (p. 2, 2007)

5.4.2 Self-Reflection or Recognizing

With the second step of ART, reflect on your options, reexamine your intentions, and reaffirm your purpose. Think about what is most important to you. Are your actions supporting your intentions? Do your actions reaffirm purpose in your life? Do your actions reaffirm purpose in your work?

Look at what you have control over and what you do not have control over. Ask yourself, "What do I need now?" (Germer and Neff 2018: 43). By simply asking the question, you allow yourself a moment of self-compassion, even if you cannot find an answer or do not have the ability to meet your needs at that time. Other ways to support yourself at work or at home include spending time with those in your support network and asking for feedback.

5.4.3 Turning Through Mindfulness

Turning, the third step of the ART Model, is about connecting to ourselves and to others. One way to do this is through mindfulness. The Greater Good Science Center at the University of California, Berkeley, shares this description of mindfulness.

"Mindfulness means maintaining a moment-by-moment awareness of our thoughts, feelings, bodily sensations, and surrounding environment, through a gentle, nurturing lens. Mindfulness also involves acceptance, meaning that we pay attention to our thoughts and feelings without judging them—without believing, for instance, that there's a 'right' or 'wrong' way to think or feel in a given moment. When we practice mindfulness, our thoughts tune into what we're sensing in the present moment rather than rehashing the past or imagining the future." (2020)

5.4.4 Examples of Mindfulness

Mindfulness can be done individually or in groups. It can be done silently, with a recording from your computer, with a phone app, in nature or a place of your choice. Below is one-minute mindful breathing exercise and a positive reminder.

5.4.4.1 One-Minute Mindful Breathing
1. Find a comfortable place to sit, placing your feet on the floor.
2. Set a timer for 1 min and gently close your eyes.
3. Breathe in through your nose and out through your mouth in an easy rhythm.

4. If thoughts arise, notice them and let them go. Relax your body as much as possible.
5. After 1 min, open your eyes and notice how you feel.

5.4.4.2 Positive Mindfulness Reminder

Another mindfulness tool you can utilize on the go is carrying a special item to remind you to become aware of your breath or slow down your heart rate. Select a word written on a piece of paper, a rock or other small item that has a positive meaning for you. Gently hold or touch the item and connect with your positive thought. As you become aware of the positive thought, focus on that good feeling for 5–10 s. Notice if this makes you feel calmer or lighter, possibly even bringing a smile to your face.

5.5   Vignette of Nurse Mindfulness-Based Drop-In Support Group

Here is an example created by the authors of connecting with both ourselves and with others in this vignette of a Nurse Mindfulness-Based Drop-In Support Group. Prior to the discussion, the nurse facilitator offered a mindful awareness practice for several minutes where the nurses noted their breath, their physical bodies, and their minds.

> *Nurse Facilitator*: Can you tell us a time in the past week you felt calm, or relaxed?
> *Nurse 1*: I did not have a time in this past week, maybe when I was asleep, but I am not sure if I was ever calm this week.
> *Nurse Facilitator*: That sounds difficult. Were you able to notice any calmness here in the group, possibly when we were doing the mindfulness practice?
> *Nurse 2*: I felt calm a few times this week when I was watching TV and not thinking about all the things I need to do.
> *Nurse 3*: I feel calm most mornings, I wake up earlier than the rest of my family. I make the coffee, then I sit down in my chair with both hands holding the cup and I feel the warmth of the cup and I smell the coffee. This is one of my favorite times of the day.
> *Nurse Facilitator*: That sounds very nice, and a great way to start your day.

5.5.1   Self-Compassion in Your Work

Self-compassion is key in connecting to ourselves and others. When you were a young child, you may have been taught the Golden Rule: "Do unto others as you would have them do unto you" (Matthew 7:12, The New King James Version Bible). You may even continue to practice this tenet in your life today. Yet, how do you treat, or speak to yourself when you have not lived up to your own expectations?

Nurses can be their own harshest critics. It may never have occurred to you to treat yourself with compassion. You might think, "I should have known that," or "Why didn't I do that?" Tara Brach states in her article *Awakening from the Trance of Unworthiness*,

"Feeling 'not good enough' is that often unseen engine that drives our daily behavior and life choices. Fear of failure and rejection feeds addictive behavior. We become trapped in workaholism – an endless striving to accomplish – and we overconsume to numb the persistent presence of fear." (2001)

This can be challenging for dedicated, caring nurses who tend to be "overachievers" and driven. You may notice you have some resistance to change even though you have identified positive changes you want to make. Be compassionate with yourself and explore why you might be resistant to change. Shaul Oreg (2003) identified six sources that may cause some people to be resistant to change—afraid of losing control, cognitive rigidity, less ability to cope with change, impatience, wanting the current structure, and preferring to keep old habits.

Self-compassion involves applying The Golden Rule to yourself; treating yourself the same way that you treat others (Dineen 2018). Ideally this includes selfcare daily as well as replacing self-judgement and self-criticism with patience and gratitude. Self-compassion is an essential skill we must learn if we are to experience sustainability and well-being in our personal life and more importantly our professional life. Self-compassion, unlike self-care, happens on the job, not off the job.

According to Christopher Germer and Kristen Neff (2013), experts in mindful self-compassion, "self-compassion is simply compassion directed inward" (p. 856). Situations come up in your life that are extremely uncomfortable. Germer and Neff go on to share (2019: 338) "when feeling overwhelmed or witnessing a painful experience, one option is to pause and say to yourself,

Everyone is on their own life journey. (pause)
I am not the cause of this person's suffering, nor is it entirely in my power to make it go away, even though I wish I could. (pause)
Moments like these are hard to witness (pause)
Yet I will help as I can."

Having an awareness of mindful self-compassion can be useful in your nursing practice. It can clarify the principles and practices of mindful self-compassion and their context in our professional nursing activities.

5.5.2 Gratitude and Compassion

In addition to self-compassion, gratitude is another way to connect to ourselves and others. Gratitude is expressing gratefulness for what is now. When you feel gratitude, you acknowledge that you are taken care of, you are not alone, and you are supported. This fills up your bucket and in turn supports you in supporting others. When you support others, you pay it forward, tapping into your sense of wealth and health, modeling a sense a spirit of generosity.

Perhaps you gratefully notice you took your break, nourishing yourself with food and drink. You might be grateful for a co-worker who helped a troubled patient, lessening the entire team's burden. Maybe it was paying attention that you arrived to work a few minutes early and you noticed the sunrise as you walked calmly into your building.

Rewire your mind for joy. Remember to pause throughout your day and notice what is happening that is right. Notice something that felt kind, friendly, or thoughtful. Wood, Froh, and Geraghty found 12 research studies supporting "the link between gratitude and subjective well-being," going on to say that "gratitude appears robustly related to mood and life satisfaction" (2010: 895). Some nurses have described themselves after acknowledging gratitude, as feeling less physically tense and having an air of lightness around them.

5.6 Connecting to Ourselves and Others, On and Off the Job

In her article "Running on Empty: Compassion Fatigue for Health Professionals" (2007), Francoise Mathieu recommends health professionals develop a Compassion Fatigue Prevention Toolkit for themselves, emphasizing this is an individual process. She gives ideas about what to include in the kit: knowing your warning signs, scheduling a regular check-in with yourself, stress relief strategies you enjoy, stress reduction strategies that work for you, and stress resiliency strategies you can use (p. 4). Cynthia Backer's FRAMES Integrative Wellness Model also supports the concept of supporting your body, mind, spirit, and emotions (2015). This model includes healthy foods, modalities to release stress, art for expression, mindfulness, energy awareness, and connection with nature through stones.

Cally Bucknell, Director of Iron County Human Services and Associates shares these steps to achieve employee well-being that appropriately apply to nurses:

Steps to Achieve Employee Well-Being
1. Set and maintain professional boundaries with colleagues and co-workers.
2. Balance your work schedule and life demands so no 1 day or 1 week is too much.
3. Make time throughout the workday for intermittent self-care breaks (i.e., lunch or afternoon walk; social time with co-workers; listen to relaxing music).
4. Create a healthy workspace for yourself.
5. Develop a short list (2–3 items) of top priorities each day.
6. Minimize procrastination and maximize a sense of control.
7. Before committing to a project, assignment or committee position, etc., first consider your needs and available resources, and whether it will lead to overextending yourself—a sure way to compromise your self-care (2019).

5.7 Conclusion: Compassion as a Nurse

Focusing on compassion for yourself and others can ultimately change the way you work as a nurse. Wherever you are in your life, it is essential to continue to cultivate compassion and care for yourself. Be patient with yourself. It takes time and continued practice to be a compassionate nurse in our complex and challenging healthcare environment. You will continue to need to address issues of pain, suffering, healthcare inequality, safety, retention, access, and time constraints relating to the volume and demands of those in need.

Contemplative practices such as self-reflection and mindfulness are skills that not only support you. They have the power to transform the way you offer nursing care. You can teach your patients and clients these simple compassionate practices and at the same time, restore yourself in healthy ways. You offer amazing care by developing and strengthening your awareness and attention to body and mind for yourself, and for others. What a wonderful opportunity for you as a nurse, to thrive, modeling healing and balance during times of stress.

> A moment of self-compassion can change your entire day. A string of such moments can change the course of your life.
> Christopher K. Germer, PhD
> *psychologist and Harvard Medical School lecturer*

Appendix 1: Extended Self-Compassion Exercise

1. Take in a few deep breaths, in through your nose, exhaling out through your mouth. Simply begin to feel your own presence, breathing in and out, at your own pace. Noting where the breath is entering, it filling your body, and exiting your body.
2. Feel the wave of movement from the inside.
3. Bring to mind someone you are caring for, someone who may be adding to your feelings of depletion.
4. Now think and feel through these sayings:
   - Everyone is on their own life journey. (pause).
   - I am not the cause of this person's suffering, nor is it entirely in my power to make it go away, even though I wish I could. (pause).
   - Moments like these are hard to witness. (pause).
   - Yet I will help as I can.
5. Again, aim to focus on your next few breaths, inhaling deeply, feeling the breath fill you, and feeling the release.
6. Allow your body to let go of tension and soften.
7. Notice your shoulders soften.
8. Notice your belly soften with each exhale.
9. Say to yourself:
   - Breath is life, without breath, there is no life.
   - My breath is supporting me.
   - Life is supporting me.

Appendix 2: What Is Meditation, and How Do I Do It?

In today's world, we are consumed with information and activity influencing our thought processes day and night. Many of us keep our electronics nearby 24 h a day. We often have constant input and it can be challenging to let down from the stimulation.

A meditation practice is a way to help you slow down, calming your mind. You let yourself simply be. There is no agenda, nothing to do, just simply pause. The goal is not to shut down your mind or your thoughts. Rather, it is to notice and be with your body. Watch your thoughts. Become aware of what your mind naturally does. A thought comes, and then the thought goes.

Mindfulness is one form of meditation. It can help you to feel rested, and more alert at the same time. You can do this sitting, lying down, walking or doing a task. Start with 1–5 min practicing this way of being with yourself, refueling yourself. The trick is to be with yourself, without judging whatever it is that you are doing. Notice and accept, without saying to yourself, "I should be….," "I wish I….," "I don't like/want….," you fill in the blank.

Appendix 3: Simple Meditation Exercise

1. Find a comfortable spot to sit.
2. Set a timer for 1–2 min and gently close your eyes.
3. Begin to notice your body.
   - What part of your body is touching the floor or the chair?
   - What is the temperature of air around you?
   - Can you smell any odors or scents?
   - Are there any sounds?
   - Can you feel or hear yourself breathe?
   - Is there any part of your body that feels tense or tight?
   - If you pay attention to the tense area, does it soften, or let go?
4. When the timer goes off, gently open your eyes, pause, and gradually move again.

Staying in this way of being for a few minutes supports your body and your mind. This can be a wonderful tool for you to practice and cultivate being with yourself.

References

American Nurses Association (ANA) (2016) American Nurses Association health risk appraisal findings. Executive summary. October 2016. https://www.nursingworld.org/~4aeeeb/globalassets/practiceandpolicy/work-environment/health%2D%2Dsafety/ana-healthriskappraisalsummary_2013-2016.pdf. Accessed 9 Jun 2020
American Nurses Association (ANA) (2020) Healthy Nurse Healthy Nation. Research. https://www.healthynursehealthynation.org/en/about/research/. Accessed 9 Jun 2020

Backer CJ (2015) FRAMES integrative wellness program for health care providers, teachers and parents. Purple Shoes Wellness. https://www.purpleshoeswellness.com/health-care-providers. Accessed 9 Jun 2020

Brach T (2001) Awakening from the trance of unworthiness. Inquiring mind. Spring 17(2). https://www.inquiringmind.com/article/1702_20_brach_awakening-from-unworthiness/

Bucknell C (2019) Steps to achieve employee well-being. Wisconsin Hawthorn Project: June 2019. https://www.wihawthornproject.com/handouts. Accessed 9 Jun 2020

Dineen F (2018) The golden rule, for yourself: the wisdom of self-compassion. Life Counseling Institute. https://lifecounselinginstitute.com/the-golden-rule-for-yourself-the-wisdom-of-self-compassion/. Accessed 9 Jun 2020

Dossey BM, Luck S, Schaub BG (2015) Appendix C-1: Integrative health and wellness assessment (short form). Nurse coaching: integrative approaches for health and wellbeing. International Nurse Coach Association, North Miami, FL, pp 434–438

Dossey BM, Luck S, Schaub BG (2015) Nurse coaching: integrative approaches for health and wellbeing. International Nurse Coach Association, North Miami, FL, pp 434–438

Germer KG, Neff KD (2013) Self-compassion in clinical practice. J Clin Pyschol 69(8):856

Germer C, Neff K (2018) The mindful self-compassion workbook. The Guilford Press, New York, NY

Germer C, Neff K (2019) Teaching the mindful self-compassion program: a guide for professionals. The Guilford Press, New York, NY

Joinson C (1992) Coping with compassion fatigue. Nursing 22(4):116–121

Kreitzer MJ, Koithan M (2019) Integrative nursing, 2nd edn. Oxford University Press, New York

Mathieu F (2007) Running on empty: compassion fatigue in health professionals. Rehab Comm Care Med:1–6

MindTools (2020) Holmes and Rahe stress scale: understanding the impact of long-term stress. https://www.mindtools.com/pages/article/newTCS_82.htm. Assessed 9 Jun 2020

Oreg S (2003) Resistance to change: developing an individual differences measure. J Appl Psychol 88(4):680

ProQOL (2020) Professional quality of measure: ProQOL measure in English and non-English translations. https://proqol.org/ProQol_Test.html. Accessed 9 Jun 2020

ProQOL Slide Set (2012) Professional quality of measure: ProQOL, compassion satisfaction, compassion fatigue, burnout and secondary traumatic stress customizable slide set. 2020. https://www.proqol.org/Customize_a_Presentation.html. Accessed 9 June 2020

Sheppard K (2016) Compassion fatigue: are you at risk? Am Nurse Today 11(1). https://www.americannursetoday.com/compassion-fatigue/. Accessed 9 Jun 2020

Skovholt TM, Trotter-Mathison M (2016) The resilient practitioner: burnout and compassion fatigue prevention and self-care strategies for the helping professions, 3rd edn. Routledge/Taylor and Francis Group, New York, NY, pp xx–xxi

Stamm B (2009). Professional quality of life: compassion satisfaction and fatigue version 5 (Proqol) 2009. Proqol.org

The Greater Good Science Center: University of California Berkeley (2020). https://greatergood.berkeley.edu/topic/mindfulness/definition. Accessed 9 Jun 2020

Todaro-Franceschi V (2019) Compassion fatigue and burnout in nursing: enhancing professional quality of life, 2nd edn. Springer, New York, NY

Wood AM, Froh JJ, Geraghty AWA (2010) Gratitude and Well-being: a review and theoretical integration. Clin Psychol Rev 30:890–905

Nutrition Strategies to Promote Wellness, Address Inadequate Nutrition, and Support Stress Reduction

6

Tanya Bachman

6.1 Introduction

Food connects humans culturally, traditionally, socially, and physically. We all need to eat to maintain our health, resulting in various food choices that we make each and every day. Because of this commonality, nutrition needs to be considered an integrative approach to individual care that is both preventative and restorative. The vitamins and minerals consumed each day are absorbed and utilized on a cellular level in every person's body. For this reason, nutrition as an integrative health strategy supports physiology and can be prescribed to positively affect each person's health in a unique way based on the individual's existing health conditions. The extent of an individual's ability to utilize nutrients is highly variable depending upon age, genetics, health, medication and substance use, and lifestyle choices (Bennett et al. 2015). However, in the case of a healthy individual, nutrition plays a tremendous role in the prevention of chronic, non-communicable diseases. Because of its role in human health, nutrition can also be part of the plan in restoring health when chronic disease does exist by defining individual risk factors such as poverty and access to healthy food, stress and trauma, activity level, age and gender, as well as psychological relationship with food.

6.2 Nutrition for Vulnerable Populations

Nutrition can serve as a first line of defense for the body. One example is that we know that nutrients like protein, vitamin C, vitamin E, vitamin D, and vitamin A all play a part in a person's immune function. When a person becomes deficient in any of these nutrients, this individual is more vulnerable to infections. In taking this a

T. Bachman (✉)
Columbia River Nutrition, Scappoose, OR, USA

© Springer Nature Switzerland AG 2021
A. Vermeesch (ed.), *Integrative Health Nursing Interventions for Vulnerable Populations*, https://doi.org/10.1007/978-3-030-60043-3_6

step further and recognizing through biochemistry knowledge that it is not just essential nutrients, but all nutrients support human health, a balanced diet will support human health. These nutrients are best obtained through a whole foods diet to provide whole vitamins, phytonutrients, and minerals to support health in addition to eliminating preservatives and other food-derived chemicals. A whole foods diet consists of fresh or frozen vegetables and fruits, whole grains like brown rice, eggs, meat, chicken, and fish. Eliminating, or significantly reducing processed foods like breads, packaged foods, candy, chips, soda, and baked goods will reduce added sugar intake and increase the nutrients consumed. This can be difficult to achieve for many people, but particularly for those in vulnerable populations experiencing food insecurity due to social determinants of health including social economic status and living in food deserts where local agriculture is not available.

In our vulnerable populations, a whole foods diet is difficult to adhere to due to cost, food storage, and food preparation. Vulnerable populations as defined by the National Collaborate Care for the Social Determinants of Health are groups and communities at a higher risk for experiencing poor health as a result of the barriers they experience to social, economic, political and environmental resources, as well as limitations due to illness or disability. These include individuals and families living in poverty, women, infants, children, elderly, immigrants, minorities, underinsured, disabled individuals, LGBTQ, HIV and AIDS positive individuals. In addition to these demographics, those with low education and literacy levels are also vulnerable because they may not understand the importance of nutrition in their health.

In looking at our vulnerable populations and access to healthy, whole food there is a tremendous potential for undernutrition to occur. For those facing socioeconomic challenges and food insecurity, not only is the cost of food a barrier but even storing and preparing food is limiting for many individuals. Often in these cases packaged food with long shelf lives and minimal food preparation requirements are preferred. In populations experiencing homelessness, this can be especially true. Lack of accessibility to healthy, whole food impacts cooking and already existing health disparities because nutrient scarcity in the daily diet exacerbates the impact of living in a state of vulnerability. Food insecurity and poor nutrition contribute to poor health outcomes including but not limited to increased risk for diabetes, cardiovascular disease, mental illness, obesity, and decreased immunity. Inadequate access to food can also set the stage for cycles of undereating and overeating, increasing the already existing stress experienced within this vulnerable population.

The current Standard American Diet puts our populations at risk for poor nutrition due to convenience, low cost, and low nutrient value of food. According to Dietary guidelines (2015), 75% of the US population is eating a diet low in fruits, vegetables, dairy, whole grains, and oils while most Americans consume too much added sugar, sodium, and saturated fat. Nutrition education can be an integrative approach to addressing food insecurity and low nutrient status in our populations. Utilizing community education through public health offices, public schools, and other community organizations can increase common knowledge of both the benefits of eating whole foods and resources to simplify the process.

6.3   Nutritional Effects on Chronic Disease

Teaching providers and patients about the importance of nourishing the body to support cellular function is vitally important to the health of our communities. Nutrition can be used to treat and manage chronic conditions, restore balance in the body, and potentially reverse certain conditions. It also provides prevention from chronic diseases. According to the CDC, 6 in 10 Americans have a chronic disease and 4 in 10 Americans have more than one chronic disease (cdc.gov/chronicdisease 2020). The CDC defines a chronic disease as "conditions that last 1 year or more and require ongoing medical attention or limit activities of daily living or both." Furthermore, the CDC states that chronic diseases are the leading causes of death and disability in the United States and are also leading drivers of the nation's $3.3 trillion in annual health care costs (cdc.gov/chronicdisease 2020). Based on that data and the crippling impact on our vulnerable populations, we need to take a more direct preventative approach using nutrition as a tool.

Using nutrition to support the body's ability to heal and restore itself is key to cut health care cost and improve population health. When individuals, families, and communities are educated to use food as a health tool, they are empowered to make changes that support their wellness. Specifically, we can utilize nutrition to support the body and potentially heal from a great variety of conditions!

Auto-immunity is a growing concern with more individuals diagnosed with an auto-immune condition each year. Additionally, it is known that auto-immunity has many connections to nutrition and gastrointestinal health (Manzel et al. 2014). Recognizing the link between the food we eat, intestinal permeability, and auto-immune prevalence can potentially help prevent and treat these conditions using food as medicine. In the United States and Western cultures, auto-immune prevalence has risen with the National Institute for Health estimating that 23.5 million Americans suffer from an auto-immune disease. The food consumed in the Western diet is high in fat, high in sugar, low in vitamins and minerals. Additionally, because the Western diet is also low in fruits and vegetables, many people are lacking antioxidant protection from inflammation. The Western diet is also high in chemicals such as preservatives, herbicides, and pesticides, potentially affecting the intestinal barrier (Visser et al. 2009). By educating communities about whole foods eating, we can potentially reduce the effects of auto-immune diseases and prevent them from occurring in some people. Without a genetic predisposition as seen in Celiac disease, the primary influence is believed to be diet. By reducing the consumption of sugar, unhealthy fats, food preservatives and increasing the consumption of whole vegetables, fruits and healthy proteins, we can provide the body with natural protection against inflammation in addition to protecting the gastrointestinal barrier from deteriorating and becoming more permeable. With increased intestinal permeability, the body will be susceptible to undigested proteins and bacteria entering the blood stream and initiating an inflammatory response systemically. Nutritional strategies to reduce these effects include: supporting a whole foods diet that is rich in fruits and vegetables, supporting a healthy gastrointestinal tract through use of fermented foods and when indicated probiotics, identifying food triggers that may initiate a breakdown in the intestinal lining, and utilizing stress reduction techniques to support vagus nerve function.

Hormone balancing, including both feeding and sex hormones, can often be obtained through nutritional strategies. All hormones are influenced by food, largely governed by hypothalamus regulation of blood sugar. Feeding hormones are negatively impacted by poor timing of meals and snacks as well as the Western diet itself, one that is rich in refined carbohydrates, chemicals, and rancid fats from its high amount of processed foods. Research shows that time restricted eating can improve insulin resistance, leptin resistance as well as improve autophagy (Longo and Panda 2016). A side effect of being a modern-day human is not only having access to food 24 h a day, but also being awake during the nighttime hours. The human circadian rhythm historically provides a time of fasting during nighttime sleeping hours, allowing the body to utilize all it has been fed during daytime hours. This is a natural way of resetting feeding hormones each night and eating when the body is experiencing true physiological hunger. Using both time restricted eating, which literally means eating between 7 a.m. and 7 p.m. with a nighttime fast, in conjunction with a whole foods diet rich in fresh produce can promote wellness in all populations with little added expense. Sex hormone are also influenced by food, as they are connected to cortisol levels. Heightened cortisol levels created by blood sugar imbalances are created predominantly by the Western diet, and can become a driver in the development of diabetes, particularly when coupled with stress (Kamba et al. 2016). With chronic high cortisol levels, the body needs to not only maintain a higher level of blood glucose, but also will begin to make less sex hormones as the need for cortisol production remains high (Whirledge and Cidlowski 2010).

This will affect reproduction and can lead to infertility due to an imbalance of sex hormones. While stress reduction is an important treatment strategy, addressing feeding behavior and foods eaten is equally important. By incorporating a whole foods diet rich in fruits and vegetables, blood sugar imbalances will be lessened and hormonal balance can be achieved in time. This 2-part strategy is universally available to all populations and is cost effective. It incorporates patient-centered treatment in addressing day to day habits and activities, empowering patients to be an intimate part of their health journey.

Chronic fatigue is a common complaint in all populations. Both a syndrome and generalized common complaint, chronic fatigue affects approximately 2.5 million Americans according to the CDC. Chronic fatigue can present as daily exhaustion that does not go away with rest, but can also present with chronic aches and pains, sleep problems, concentration problems, and difficulty restoring energy after exertion. This type of fatigue puts people at risk for additional health-related problems due to the simple lack of energy. How can one adopt a healthy lifestyle that includes healthy eating and exercise when he/she can hardly get through the day and sometimes even struggles with getting out of bed? Nutrition can work as an integrative health strategy to support the body and heal from chronic fatigue. When considering all that is lacking in the Western diet, it becomes clear that many of those struggling with chronic fatigue are most likely nutrient deficient. While random control trials have not been done extensively to support the use of nutrient therapy in chronic fatigue, observational evidence may tell us differently. When testing chronic fatigue patients for nutrient deficiencies, they respond well to nutrient therapy (Castro-Marrero et al. 2017). When testing for nutrient insufficiencies in the US population, one study showed persons to commonly be "below the estimated average requirement for vitamins A (35%), C (31%), D (74%), and E (67%) as well as calcium (39%) and magnesium (46%)" (Wallace et al. 2014). While this is not an area of great research using RTCs, it is reasonable to approach chronic fatigue using nutritional strategies considering the role nutrients play in cellular health. In mitochondrial function, specific minerals are necessary to make ATP (adenosine triphosphate) and when they are not present, ATP production diminishes. Specifically, we need a B vitamin complex, but especially B1, B2, B3, zinc, manganese, and magnesium in addition to L-carnitine which is needed to shuttle fat between cells. When we consider the role of mitochondria in energy and the micronutrient support needed for mitochondrial function, it becomes clear that nutrition plays a role in generalized fatigue and chronic fatigue in humans. Without the cellular capacity to create ATP, people will present with low energy levels. This coupled with high stress in our vulnerable populations where stress contributes to enhanced mineral deficiency and imbalanced blood sugar leads to communities struggling with energy. Using whole foods nutrition can easily provide needed nourishment to support ATP production and potentially increase energy levels in vulnerable populations and all populations.

Diabetes is well known to be affected by nutrition and stress. Diabetes continues to prevail in the USA, but particularly in vulnerable populations experiencing high stress, food insecurity, and lower socioeconomic levels. Foods that are inexpensive and convenient in the Western diet also are known to be nutrient lacking, starving the body of necessary vitamins and minerals. These foods support the onset of type 2 diabetes in many ways, including reducing healthy fats in the diet that support cellular and mitochondrial health, reducing healthy protein in the diet that promotes satiety, creating a high sugar load on the pancreas in turn affecting insulin signaling, and negatively affecting the health of the gut microbiome. Research has shown that alterations in the gut microbiome are related to foods eaten and in cases of diabetes, there are reductions in beneficial bacteria that are anti-inflammatory, while simultaneously there are increases in harmful bacteria that promote inflammation (Meghan 2016). Foods that support beneficial bacteria are whole foods such as fruits, vegetables, whole grains, lean meat, nuts, and seeds. These are not foods commonly associated with the Western diet, and when comparing nutrient density of the Western diet and a whole foods diet, it is clear how type 2 diabetes develops. When cellular health is not supported through a whole foods diet, rich in micronutrients, healthy fat, fiber, carbohydrate, and lean protein, cellular health declines and sets the stage for insulin resistance. Looking at the influence of a whole foods diet on insulin and blood sugar, research shows that the prebiotic fiber found in whole foods like fruits, vegetables, legumes, and whole grains not only fees beneficial gut microbes, but improves satiety, thus decreasing food intake (Meghan 2016). These create reduced postprandial glucose levels, serving to support insulin sensitivity. Insulin sensitivity is the prevailing issue in type 2 diabetes and can be restored through eating a whole foods diet rich in cell supporting nutrients. For individuals experiencing food insecurity, insulin resistance is heightened in part due to the utilization of inexpensive, nutrient dense foods that are high in calories but also due to the effects of stress and feeding hormones that are part of the cycle of food insecurity (Lopez and Seligman 2012). Food insecurity enhances hypoglycemic and hyperglycemic states in the body as nutritious foods are not easily obtained and times of going without food at all reduce the positive, balancing effects of a nourished body. Recognizing these challenges, the United States needs to incorporate policy change, targeting vulnerable populations experiencing food insecurity. Homes with children, particularly those with a single income, experience greater health disparities linked to food insecurity. Programs that can support families and individuals experiencing food insecurity can have a tremendous impact on health outcomes related to type 2 diabetes and its comorbidities. By utilizing whole foods to support the body's blood sugar balancing and insulin sensitivity, communities can experience wellness and improved quality of living. Struggling with diabetes in a food insecure environment only increases the incidence of comorbidities like cardiovascular disease and peripheral neuropathy. Educating communities about the benefits and ease of a whole foods diet plan provides a tool box to empower individuals in their health journey.

Cardiovascular disease closely linked to the long-term effects of diabetes can be not only positively influenced by diet, but potentially reversed in some individuals. Statistics clearly tell us that cardiovascular disease is a comorbidity of type 2 diabetes and that both are related to diet. In a recent research meta-analysis, it was found that "Globally, overall CVD affects approximately 32.2% of all persons with T2DM. CVD is a major cause of mortality among people with T2DM, accounting for approximately half of all deaths over the study period. Coronary artery disease and stroke were the major contributors." (Einarson et al. 2018). Cardiovascular disease alone accounts for 1 in 4 deaths in the United States (cdc.gov/chronicdisease 2020). These are mostly preventable deaths, as cardiovascular disease is very closely related to diet. The underlying mechanism in cardiovascular disease is endothelial damage caused by system inflammation that is directly related to dietary sources like unhealthy fats, refined sugar, and a lack of antioxidants provided by fresh fruits and vegetables (Widmer and Lerman 2014). The Westernized diet is a social driver in CVD for those in vulnerable populations and for busy working people. Using nutritional nudges (simple, usable nutrition and healthy eating tips) in the community setting can heighten the awareness of healthy eating and how attainable it can be for people struggling to eat healthy. Educational tools like patient handouts and simple healthy eating classes at community health centers, healthy eating classes at local schools, churches and public health centers are ways to engage community members in ways to eat to support their health. The heart as a vital organ responds quite well to nutritional strategies, and helping individuals identify foods that support a healthy heart in addition to foods that increase inflammation and damage the heart can change the health of our communities. Added to this, incorporating information about how to cook healthy foods and where to obtain them relatively inexpensively is necessary to include all members within a community. Community food pantries and farmer's markets are available in most areas and provide fresh, nourishing foods that support cardiovascular health. Utilizing pantries for vulnerable members of communities is important to include them in these efforts to promote wellness in all populations. Farmer's markets often provide fresh produce at a fraction of the cost compared to grocery stores, plus the produce is locally obtained and rich in nutrients for added nourishment.

Clearly nutrition information can be an easily obtained tool for patients and practitioners alike in battling the ongoing effects of chronic disease. The added bonus is there are not negative health outcomes in supporting the body through nourishment. For individuals facing advanced effects of chronic disease, the added nutrients can only serve to improve quality of life and overall management of any given chronic disease.

6.4   Nutrition at the Community Level

Eating healthy, nourishing food is a powerful way to improve the health of communities. It takes education, commitment, and inclusion of all community members to ensure everyone is aware of resources within a given community that provide healthy foods. These resources are frequently found through pantries, community kitchens, farmer's markets, home gardens, seed sharing, and community gardens in addition to services like Women, Infants, and Children (WIC), school hot meal programs, and Supplemental Nutrition Assistance Programs (SNAP).

Depending upon the region, pantries often partner with state food banks to provide food for those experiencing food insecurity. In Oregon, community pantries partner with the Oregon Food Bank, allowing pantries to provide a variety of nourishing foods that are often donated by local farmers and grocery stores. This partnership provides vulnerable community members with locally grown fresh produce that is freely given highly encouraged at pantry sites in every neighborhood. Some pantries are home to a soup kitchen or community kitchen which adds to the availability of nourishing foods for struggling community members. It is a place of gathering, warmth, and support within a community which can lessen the effects of stress associated with the social determinants of health.

Community gardens, seed sharing, and home gardening are added resources that provide communities with nourishing whole foods. As cities grow and green spaces shrink, often one will find an area in a neighborhood set aside as a community garden. This is a place where healthy foods can be grown and shared with community members. While it may take more resources to grow a personal garden, when sharing space within a community and sharing the harvest, community members are engaged in healthy activity and in healthy eating. Additionally, when using the harvest to share in the creation of healthy dishes and canning soups, sauces and salsas, a community is nourished not just physically, but on an interpersonal and spiritual level.

Government programs like WIC, public school hot lunch/breakfast, and SNAP also work to provide nourishing foods to vulnerable populations. Awareness of these programs, how they work, and where they can be found for community members is important when providing patient care and patient education in a variety of settings. While screening for poverty and food insecurity, ensuring that individuals and families know where to seek support through programs like these is vital to including all community members in their own wellness. Without hot lunch programs, many children will not eat a meal during the day and without WIC, families may have less access to protein rich, nourishing foods.

There are additional challenges to face when working with nutrition as a health promotion strategy. Working hours, education level, belief in nutrition as a wellness tool, stress, motivation, and self-belief all factor in. There are many strategies that can be used to help individuals create healthy habits that support weekly healthy eating!

An individual's working hours is potentially one of the top reasons people choose unhealthy foods. It is unarguable that eating a healthy, whole foods diet requires time in the kitchen. This is time that not everyone is willing to spend or feels they have the energy to spend after a long day at work. The convenience of packaged foods, pre-prepared foods, and fast foods are alluring in this scenario. Using nutrition classes to teach community members about strategies for simple meals and meal preparation can help them overcome this obstacle. Specific strategies include weekend meal prepping and cooking large amounts to freeze for later use. It can seem overwhelming for anyone working full time to go home and prepare a meal at the end of a long day! Teaching individuals how to make food ahead on a weekend can help tremendously. This might include washing and chopping vegetables and fruit, pre-cooking rice or quinoa, pre-cooking meats like chicken and hamburger, and pre-cooking meals like soups and sauces on the weekends in large amounts for storage and use throughout the week. Creating a habit to make twice as much when cooking a meal will provide freezer options for a later time.

6.5 Nutrition and Stress

Stress is also a factor that contributes to unhealthy food choices. People in a stressed state may not feel they have the time to dedicate to cooking and meal prep, and therefore rely on convenience food instead. Added to this, chronic stress alters human hormones and leaves one in a state of high cortisol levels. Chronically elevated cortisol levels are known to create imbalanced blood sugars and have been found to be linked to an increased risk in type 2 diabetes (Joseph and Golden 2017). Vulnerable populations faced not only with high day to day stress but also limited resources to purchase AND prepare healthy, whole foods are at an even higher risk for developing type 2 diabetes and its comorbidities. This is a cycle seen in communities facing various socioeconomic challenges has been researched more in depth in recent years. Findings are telling, supporting not only nutrition as a tool to reduce disease risk, but also supporting the need for stress reduction techniques being taught and used by community members.

Mind body medicine has varying effects on human physiology, its most important one for this discussion being its ability to reduce stress hormones and restore blood pressure, heart rate, and respiration rate in most people (Brower 2006). Because many mind body modalities are cost free and therefore accessible to everyone, they are additional tools that can be used in vulnerable communities affected by high stress hormones in relation to social determinants of health. Modalities like Yoga, tai chi, deep breathing, visualization, music therapy, and guided meditation are easily found and can be used anywhere. Many of these modalities can be used to strengthen both family and community bonds, encouraging a deeper sense of resilience in vulnerable populations. For example, partnering with a community center to provide free beginner Yoga classes or meditation classes gives community members a place to participate and fellow community members to collaborate with. In such settings, it is also not uncommon to see food pantries open several days a week. These spaces can provide opportunities to support all members of a community, ensuring nutrition, stress, and a sense of belonging are all addressed. These are integrative health strategies that are simple yet powerful ways that communities can be supported in ways that can improve health outcomes. These strategies can be set in place by community organizers, health educators, and public health professionals like nurses and with community partnerships can provide years of community health support for all members of a community.

6.6   Conclusion

When using existing community resources to grow programs centered around positive health outcomes, possibilities are endless. Not only are direct challenges like food insecurity and social determinants of health addressed, personal challenges are also addressed. Overcoming one's education level, and building motivation and self-belief can come from developing integrative health programs in vulnerable communities. There are many other difficult circumstances faced by community members that add to the level of stress and personal choices such as addiction, adverse childhood experiences, and interpersonal violence that can be helped with community centers focused on integrative health measures discussed in this chapter. Taking time to work in vulnerable populations and teach individuals about healthy choices beginning with food can build self-belief and help people feel better. The better we feel, the more motivated most of us are to continue fostering self-care.

References

Bennett BJ et al (2015) Nutrition and the science of disease prevention: a systems approach to support metabolic health. Ann N Y Acad Sci 1352:1–12. Accessed 1 Jun 2020. https://doi.org/10.1111/nyas.12945

Brower V (2006) Mind-body research moves towards the mainstream. EMBO Rep 7(4):358–361. Accessed 1 Jun 2020. https://doi.org/10.1038/sj.embor.7400671

Castro-Marrero J et al (2017) Treatment and management of chronic fatigue syndrome/myalgic encephalomyelitis: all roads lead to Rome. Br J Pharmacol 174(5):345–369. Accessed 1 Jun 2020. https://doi.org/10.1111/bph.13702

cdc.gov/chronicdisease (2020). https://www.cdc.gov/chronicdisease/about/index.htm. Accessed 1 Jun 2020

Dietary Guidelines (2015). https://health.gov/dietaryguidelines/2015/guidelines/chapter-2/current-eating-patterns-in-the-united-states/. Accessed 1 Jun 2020

Einarson T et al (2018) Prevalence of cardiovascular disease in type 2 diabetes: a systematic literature review of scientific evidence from across the world in 2007–2017. Cardiovasc Diabetol 17:83. Accessed 1 Jun 2020

Joseph JJ, Golden SH (2017) Cortisol dysregulation: the bidirectional link between stress, depression, and type 2 diabetes mellitus. Ann N Y Acad Sci 1391(1):20–34. Accessed 1 Jun 2020. https://doi.org/10.1111/nyas.13217

Kamba A et al (2016) Association between higher serum cortisol levels and decreased insulin secretion in a general population. PLoS One 11(11):e0166077. Accessed 1 Jun 2020. https://doi.org/10.1371/journal.pone.0166077

Longo VD, Panda S (2016) Fasting, circadian rhythms, and time-restricted feeding in healthy lifespan. Cell Metab 23(6):1048–1059. Accessed 1 Jun 2020. https://doi.org/10.1016/j.cmet.2016.06.001

Lopez A, Seligman H (2012) Clinical management of food-insecure individuals with diabetes. Diabetes Spectr 25(1):14–18. Accessed 1 Jun 2020. https://doi.org/10.2337/diaspect.25.1.14

Manzel A et al (2014) Role of "Western diet" in inflammatory autoimmune diseases. Curr Allergy Asthma Rep 14(1):404. https://doi.org/10.1007/s11882-013-0404-6

Meghan J (2016) Nutrition considerations for microbiota health in diabetes. Diabetes Spectr 29(4):238–244. Accessed 1 Jun 2020. https://doi.org/10.2337/ds16-0003

Visser J et al (2009) Tight junctions, intestinal permeability, and autoimmunity: celiac disease and type 1 diabetes paradigms. Ann N Y Acad Sci 1165:195–205. Accessed 1 Jun 2020. https://doi.org/10.1111/j.1749-6632.2009.04037.x

Wallace TC et al (2014) Multivitamin/mineral supplement contribution to micronutrient intakes in the United States, 2007–2010. J Am Coll Nutr 33(2):94–102. Accessed 1 Jun 2020. https://doi.org/10.1080/07315724.2013.846806

Whirledge S, Cidlowski JA (2010) Glucocorticoids, stress, and fertility. Minerva Endocrinol 35(2):109–125. Accessed 1 Jun 2020

Widmer RJ, Lerman A (2014) Endothelial dysfunction and cardiovascular disease. Glob Cardiol Sci Pract 2014(3):291–308. Accessed Jun 1 2020

Working with Community Populations to Increase Wellness

7

Barbara J. Braband

7.1 Introduction

Community populations present a rich context to optimize wellness where we live, work, and recreate in groups. Based on a broader definition of health that embraces wellness, the majority of healthcare delivery is transitioning beyond clinics and hospitals into community settings. Many advantages for targeting the delivery of population-focused integrative healthcare services include the expanded social relationships through familial, economic, social, and faith-based connections rather than the limited individual perspective. Health and wellness behaviors and outcomes are influenced through these natural social connections where people invest their lives and work. Levels of trust and bonds with one another either positively or negatively influence health behavior choices and outcomes. This chapter will explore the evidence for integrative health nursing interventions aimed at the community.

Interventions directed at this crucial point of care in communities offer upstream, preventive advantages to reduce health risks and maximize health benefits for groups rather than individuals. One case example highlighting the benefits of population-focused preventive community programs compared to an individualized approach comes from Iceland. The adolescent population in Iceland experienced an epidemic level of dangerous levels of binge drinking in the late 1970s, 1980s, and early 1990s. Preventive programs in Iceland for alcohol and drug education were implemented targeting many areas of the adolescents' lives through community and family-oriented interventions. These areas included organized leisure activities like sports offered three to four times a week resulting in reduced unsupervised free time and negative effects of peer group pressure; more time spent with parents to enhance parental control and connection; school programs that promoted mental health; and

B. J. Braband (✉)
School of Nursing, University of Portland, Portland, OR, USA
e-mail: braband@up.edu

© Springer Nature Switzerland AG 2021
A. Vermeesch (ed.), *Integrative Health Nursing Interventions for Vulnerable Populations*, https://doi.org/10.1007/978-3-030-60043-3_7

parental education related to the negative effects of peer pressure on drinking behavior (Kristjansson et al. 2009). Parental involvement played a critical role in curbing adolescent drinking in Iceland. This study noted the decline of adolescent alcohol abstainers [among adolescents aged 15–16] in Iceland grew from "20.8% in 1995 to 65.5% in 2015" (Nordic Welfare Center 2019). One way that parents intervened included their efforts to patrol neighborhoods to talk to young people who were outside late at night and urge them to go home (Kristjansson et al. 2016). These community programs highlight action, with an emphasis on control, at many levels of community involvement. In summary, when community resources and activities were implemented in response to this epidemic over several decades of intensive community intervention programs, the incidence of teen drinking declined in Iceland (Nordic Welfare Center 2019).

7.2   Expanded Perspectives for Integrative Health

Historically, integrative health interventions and programs have been based on a limited definition of health, but a broader definition of health is emerging extending care "beyond the clinic to society at large" (Wit et al. 2017). Wit et al. (2017) reported on an updated definition, following review by more than 200 researchers, clinicians, and medical educators with additional input from several integrative health organizations including the Academic Consortium of Integrative Medicine and Health and the International Society for Complementary Medicine Research (Wit et al. 2017: 135, Fig. 7.1):

> Integrative Health is a state of well-being in body, mind, and spirit that reflects aspects of the individual, community, and population. It is affected by: (1) individual biological factors and behaviors, social values, and public policy, (2) the physical, social, and economic environments, and (3) an integrative healthcare system that involves the active participation of the individual and the healthcare team in applying a broad spectrum of

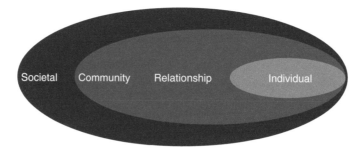

Fig. 7.1 The Social Ecological Model: A Framework for Prevention. (Source: https://www.cdc.gov/violenceprevention/images/X-social-ecologicalmodel.jpg)

preventive and therapeutic approaches. Integrative health encourages individuals, social groups, and communities to develop ways of being that promote meaning, resilience, and wellbeing across the life course (p. 135, Fig. 7.1).

This definition addressed eight primary domains as follows:

1. inter-relationships among all health-related domains;
2. the role of health determinants outside of healthcare (e.g., personal behaviors, genetics);
3. the role of upstream determinants (e.g., physical and social environment);
4. empowerment of individuals, groups, and communities;
5. the value of person-centered, evidence-based care;
6. receipt of appropriate services;
7. community-based strategies;
8. population-based strategies (Wit et al. 2017: 135).

As this definition of integrative health continues to expand, the recognition of the critical role of community and population-based strategies resonates with further momentum. An urgency exists at the heart of integrative health promotion, targeting an upstream awareness of the impact of health determinants, for health across the lifespan.

The demand for integrative health services, along with fair and equitable payment mechanisms, is growing as individuals explore these services and experience positive health outcomes contributing to their own wellness. Advantageous strategies to reach more individuals, families, and organizations can be achieved through population-focused planning, assessment, interventions, and evaluation of integrative healthcare programs. If integrative health services expand their utilization of community and population-based strategies to improve health and prevent disease, wellness can be optimized for a broader sector of our populations in considerably less time at a potentially lower cost than relying on an individualized approach for these services (Wit et al. 2017).

7.3 Population-Focused Community Concepts

What does community-based population-focused healthcare consist of? What are the primary concepts and interventions that could guide a broader implementation of integrative healthcare? Let us consider the following concepts as we explore how to advance the delivery of integrative healthcare to the level of population-focused interventions and programs.

According to Espina et al. (2016), "effective, evidence-based public health practices focused at a population level are needed to reform health systems and reduce health disparities." Key concepts related to population health include health promotion, health prevention, the social-ecological framework, social determinants of health, community-academic partnerships, and community-based participatory research (CBPR) with key community stakeholders. Please refer to Table 7.1 the Population-focused Community Concepts Toolkit to guide your concept review.

Population health. First, population health is defined as "a larger group whose members may or may not interact with one another but who share at least one characteristic such as age, gender, ethnicity, residence, or a shared health issue" such as diabetes or hypertension (Savage et al. 2016: 10; Kindig and Stoddart 2003). In

Table 7.1 Population-focused Community Concepts Toolkit

Concept	Definition	Examples
Population	"A larger group whose members may or may not interact with one another but who share at least one characteristic such as age, gender, ethnicity, residence, or a shared health issue" (Savage et al. 2016: 16).	One population would be prenatal mothers and fathers within a primary clinic.
Community	"A group of individuals living within the same geographic area, such as a town or a neighborhood, or a group of individuals who share some other common denominator, such as ethnicity or religious orientation" (Savage et al. 2016: 10). It is similar to a population, but a key difference is the level of social interaction or relationships with community members.	Community members often share decision-making. One community example would be a group of prenatal parents who attend childbirth classes and get acquainted, lend peer support, and extend interactions to shared play groups and child-care exchanges.
Health promotion	"The process of enabling people to increase control over, and to improve, their health" (WHO 1998).	Examples include a broad range of healthcare services that enhance control and improve health through access to services, education, and self-management for all aspects of health not limited to nutrition, sleep, exercise, and environment.
Risk reduction or health protection	According to WHO (1998), *risk reduction* refers to "actions taken to reduce a person's risk for disease," while *health protection* focuses on enhancing the person's ability to guard against disease (Savage et al. 2016).	*Risk reduction* behaviors that limit disease risk include overall healthy behaviors and routines like daily exercise, bike helmet safety, and yoga. Examples of *health protection* programs would offer individuals vaccines, diets, or stress management activities to target specific diseases.
Ecological or community Health promotion	Population-level terms used in reference to health promotion (Savage et al. 2016).	Integrative health examples include persons in a community with chronic depression who benefit from targeted advocacy and coaching programs to better manage stress with integrative health treatments such as yoga, reiki, and massage.

Table 7.1 (continued)

Concept	Definition	Examples
Health prevention and levels of prevention	Interventions that reduce risks or threats to optimal health. This includes the prevention of disease and injury as well as limiting the progress of related diseases or health conditions (Savage et al. 2016). There are three primary levels of prevention: (a) Primary—Upstream interventions targeting persons at risk for disease or injury *before it occurs;* (b) Secondary—Interventions that strive to detect the disease or injury early through screening and assessment to initiate prompt effective treatment before secondary complications or other limitations occur; (c) Tertiary—Prevention of long-term disability through rehabilitative interventions to prevent premature death (Institute for Work and Health 2017).	An ecological example is based on an environmental exposure when chemicals are discharged in a river upstream from a community. *Primary prevention:* Community members pursue prompt action to stop the company from this chemical discharge practice to remove the hazardous exposure. *Secondary prevention:* If the chemical exposure goes undetected, screening persons who swam in the river and now have rashes will alert the community to this issue. Affected individuals will need to receive prompt treatment. *Tertiary prevention:* If swimmers' rashes go undetected and/or untreated, or if swimmers continue to swim in the river, community programs may need to address finding alternative safe swimming sites and additional treatments and policies.
Social-ecological framework	This framework guides the assessment and implementation of all levels of care including individuals, relationships with families and organizations, community, and society (see Fig. 7.1) (IOM 2003a; CDC 2019).	Refer to Fig. 7.1 for the Social Ecological Model: A Framework for Prevention Model (CDC 2019). Examples illustrate connections between all levels of care for various health concerns. An elderly person (individual) lives in an assisted care setting with no family nearby (relationships and institutions), but her community offers a volunteer respite program with weekly visitors (community) in a society that regulates elder care and outreach programs.
Social determinants of health	"Conditions in the environment in which people are born, live, learn, work, play, worship, and age that affect a wide range of health, functioning, and quality-of-life outcomes and risks" (Institute of Medicine 2002; Healthy People 2020a).	Healthy People 2020 offers a place-based framework that recognizes five primary social determinants of health: neighborhood and built environment; health and healthcare; social and community context; education; and economic stability (see Fig. 7.2).

(continued)

Table 7.1 (continued)

Concept	Definition	Examples
Academic-community partnerships	These partnerships between academic institutional settings and programs with formal community organizations and/or informal community groups, leaders, and stakeholders create pathways beyond traditional healthcare settings (Healthy People 2020b; Kulbok et al. 2015; Hassouneh et al. 2011) to maximize health promotion outcomes.	Community settings that often affiliate with academic partners include nursing centers, housing developments, neighborhood centers, parishes, school health programs, and occupational health programs that target high-risk vulnerable populations such as the frail elderly, homeless persons, teen mothers, and all persons and groups at risk for health issues.
Community-based participatory research (CBPR)	A primary collaborative research approach that is often embedded within community-based partnerships "to enhance partnerships and empower community members as participants by including them in the decision-making processes of assessment and program planning" (Andrews et al. 2007; Hassouneh et al. 2011; Perry and Hoffman 2010).	CBPR projects can offer students in academic programs, such as integrative health, combined practicum and formal research experiences that foster integrative health promotion in areas not limited to nutrition, stress management, health prevention, and health education community outreach activities.

contrast, a community is similar in some respects, but a key difference is the level of social interaction or relationships with members of that community who often share decision-making. Savage et al. (2016) define a community as "a group of individuals living within the same geographical area, such as a town or a neighborhood, or a group of individuals who share some other common denominator, such as ethnicity or religious orientation" (p. 10). One community example includes a group of prenatal parents from one primary clinic who attend the same childbirth class and get acquainted with each other, lend peer support to one another, and extend these interactions to shared play groups and child-care exchanges.

Health promotion and risk reduction or health protection. These concepts are intertwined, yet discrete concepts that limit disease occurrence or its severity, to promote optimal health and wellness. According to the World Health Organization (WHO 1998), **health promotion** is characterized as the "process of enabling people to increase control over, and to improve, their health." Savage et al. (2016) propose the updated term of **health protection** to replace **risk reduction** characterized as "actions taken to reduce a person's risk for disease (WHO 1998)," contrasting the new term with a focus on enhancing the person's ability to guard against disease. An example of risk reduction behaviors that limit disease risk includes overall healthy behaviors and routines like daily exercise, bike helmet safety, and yoga while a health protection example could include offering individuals specific vaccines, diets, or stress management activities to address specific diseases. Savage et al. note that the term, health promotion, when directed at a population level is often referred to as **ecological health promotion** or **community health promotion**. According to Kok et al. (2008), ecological health promotion is directed toward environmental change through community stakeholders and members who work toward the implementation of change in their communities. Racher and Annis (2008) propose a community action model summarizing how these population-level health promotion perspectives collectively engage persons in community-oriented problem-solving, empowerment, political change, and environmental enhancement rather than an individualized approach based on lifestyle and behavioral changes. Integrative health examples include persons in a community with chronic depression who benefit from targeted advocacy and coaching programs to better manage stress with integrative health treatments such as yoga, Reiki, acupuncture, or massage.

Health prevention and levels of prevention. Health prevention is a broad concept in population health referring to interventions that reduce risks or threats to optimal health. According to Savage et al. (2016), health prevention includes the prevention of disease and injury, as well as the progression of related diseases or health conditions. A traditional public health approach or framework to prevention based on the natural disease progression is the **levels of prevention** model. According to the Institute for Work and Health (2017), three levels of prevention guide health promotion interventions: *primary prevention* includes upstream interventions targeting persons at risk for disease or injury before it occurs. The upstream approach is aimed at interventions to limit the potential causes of disease or injury, such as environmental or economic threats, that elevate an individual or population's risk for disease or injury. Examples include policies that mandate safe and healthy practices like bike helmets or safety belts. *Secondary prevention* interventions strive to detect the disease or injury early through screening and assessment to initiate prompt effective treatment before secondary complications or other health limitations occur. Exercise programs that limit the impact of cardiovascular disease or work modifications for injured or ill workers are examples for secondary levels of prevention. Finally, *tertiary health prevention* is focused on the prevention of long-term disability through rehabilitation interventions, such as stroke recovery programs, to prevent premature death. An ecological example of these levels of prevention is based on a situation when chemicals are discharged in a river upstream from a community. If community members pursue prompt action to stop the company from this practice to remove the hazardous exposure, you have accomplished primary prevention. However, if the exposure goes undetected or is not stopped, swimmers in the river may develop serious and persistent rashes. Secondary prevention is accomplished when the swimmers' rashes are screened and treated promptly and effectively. But if swimmers' rashes are not detected promptly or swimmers continue to swim in the river, a tertiary prevention option may include setting up community programs to teach swimmers how to live with their persistent rashes by limiting the impact of the rash or where they might seek alternative sites for swimming. Most health issues are best addressed with a combination of the three levels of prevention, with the greatest impact when problems are completely avoided with primary prevention, or when issues are detected early by secondary prevention practices (Institute for Work and Health 2017).

Social-ecological framework. The social-ecological framework has been a leading emerging public health framework to guide the assessment and implementation of all levels of care in response to the Institute of Medicine (IOM) report in 2003. The initial report, The *Future of the Public's Health in the Twenty-First Century*

(Institute of Medicine 2003a), supported the implementation of the social ecological model that recognizes how health is influenced at various social levels. The IOM (2003b) distinguishes the framework as "a model of health that emphasizes linkages and relationships among multiple factors (or determinants) affecting health." The model includes levels of linkages including individuals, relationships or interpersonal levels, community (including institutional environments), and society (that encompasses broader social, economic, and political influences) (Refer to Fig. 7.1: The social ecological model: A framework for prevention model) (CDC 2019). A common application for this ecological framework is obesity with a limited list of potential examples to follow. Individual factors impacting obesity cover a wide array including genetics, epigenetics, as well as knowledge, attitudes, and behaviors surrounding diet and exercise. At the interpersonal or relationship level, cultural factors like traditions, cultural meanings of being thin or fat, and food choices are prominent. Community applications often focus on norms for food choices, food access and affordability as well as access to exercise facilities and outdoor spaces while institutional factors connect with school and workplace food options and exercise opportunities. Finally, community-level factors promote regulations, offer food subsidies, and guide food packaging and food safety issues.

Social determinants of health. The social-ecological framework is also impacted by the **social determinants of health,** defined as conditions in the environment in which people are born, live, learn, work, play, worship, and age that affect a wide range of health, functioning, and quality-of-life outcomes and risks. Contextual conditions (e.g., social, economic, and physical) in these various environments and settings (e.g., school, church, workplace, and neighborhood) have been referred to as "place" (IoM 2002; Healthy People 2020a). Healthy People 2020 offers a place-based framework for five primary social determinants of health including: neighborhood and built environment, health and healthcare, social and community context, education, and economic stability (refer to Fig. 7.2). These social determinants of health provide a comprehensive context to examine the primary issues challenging the attainment of health equity. Our current healthcare system is undergoing extensive reform to embrace a commitment to an "ecological and determinants approach to health promotion and disease prevention" (p. 2, Healthy People 2020a: Framework) in its new overarching goal to "create social and physical environments that promote health for all" (p. 1).

The U.S. Department of Health and Human Services, in the Healthy People 2030: Framework (n.d.), has placed an increased emphasis on addressing equitable health for communities according to the first foundational principle of the framework, "health and well-being of all people and communities are essential to a thriving, equitable society." "Creating social and physical environments that promote good health for all" has been one of the four primary goals of Healthy People 2020 for the past decade (Healthy People 2020a).

Academic and community-based partnerships support health promotion to optimize wellness. **Academic and community-based partnerships and community-based participatory research (CBPR)** present clinical (or practicum) contextual

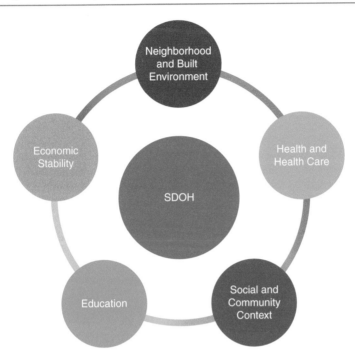

Fig. 7.2 Social Determinants of Health. (Source: https://www.healthypeople.gov/sites/default/files/styles/featured_image_on_topic_page/public/2020/topicsobjectives2020/images/SDOH_m.png?itok=qU7E8Stf)

opportunities to foster and test implementation strategies for integrative healthcare in communities. Academic partnerships in community-based programs create pathways to reach persons beyond traditional healthcare settings including schools, worksites, healthcare facilities, and communities (Healthy People 2020b). These partnerships maximize health promotion outcomes through reduced investment of time and resources by working through existing social structures where pre-existing peer social interactions can foster sharing of heath information and interventions. The goals of these partnerships consist of creating collaborative partnerships with community leaders and stakeholders and identifying resources and solutions to problems through community-based participatory research (CBPR) methods (Kulbok et al. 2015; Hassouneh et al. 2011). Potential examples of these partnerships include nursing centers, housing developments, neighborhood centers, parishes, school health programs, and occupational health programs that target high-risk vulnerable populations such as frail elderly, homeless persons, teen mothers, and anyone at risk for a specific disease. Key characteristics that foster development of an effective collaborative community-based partnership relationship emerged based on a retrospective case study of a long-term academic and community-based partnership over 7 years within one academic program and a nearby local community garden and market program. These four key characteristics included the: "(a) development of a joint mission and strategic plan; (b) a partnership structure with clear expectations, roles, and communication channels at all partnership levels;

c) increased duration of engagement to allow for meaningful learning experiences and community benefits; and d) adequate and shared leadership, accountability, resources, and rewards between organizations" (Mayer et al. 2017). A foundation of strong collaboration can open doors to sustainable educational opportunities for students and innovations to address key health problems in communities.

Community-based participatory research (CBPR) is a primary research approach often embedded within these academic and community-based partnerships "to enhance partnerships and empower community members as participants by including them in the decision-making processes of assessment and program planning" (Andrews et al. 2007; Hassouneh et al. 2011; Perry and Hoffman 2010). CBPR is a collaborative research approach characterized by sustainable partnerships between academic and community stakeholders to explore and implement multiple levels of culturally centered interventions based on an ecological framework with individuals, groups, organizations, and communities (Kulbok et al. 2015; Sandoval et al. 2012).

Public health nursing has evolved to address these community dimensions of practice that may also guide and support the implementation of integrative health interventions within communities and populations. Kulbok et al. (2015) note three primary competencies that can be incorporated with CBPR methods. The first competency includes analytic assessment to support health promotion and prevention for complex community health challenges by hearing multiple voices from community insiders. These "community voices" may include stakeholders, advisory boards, and community health workers (CHWs). A cultural competency domain helps healthcare personnel understand "invisible factors in the community that promote health and prevent disease, such as assets, values, strengths, and special characteristics of the communities" (Kulbok et al. 2015; Anderson and McFarlane 2011). Finally, program planning competence can "develop sustainable programs and build community capacity for health promotion by taking into account the ecological context of the community from an ethnographic assessment" (Kulbok et al. 2015). According to the Quad Council of Public Health Nurses (2011), additional community-based health promotion skills and competencies include "communication, financial planning and management, leadership and systems thinking, policy development, and public health science."

The measurement of health outcomes of CBPR studies that benefit communities presents particular challenges based on the complexity of measuring CBPR pathways of change within academic-community collaborations. Despite the promising benefits of CBPR studies to promote health in communities, gaps remain in how CBPR processes work and how the success of partnerships is evaluated (Sandoval et al. 2012). A systematic evaluation study was conducted to assess existing measures of the four components of CBPR Conceptual Model first proposed by Wallerstein et al. (2008), with subsequent adaptations by Wallerstein and Duran (2010). The model's four primary core components include contexts, group dynamics processes (individual, relational, and structural), intervention/research design, and outcomes (see Fig. 7.3).

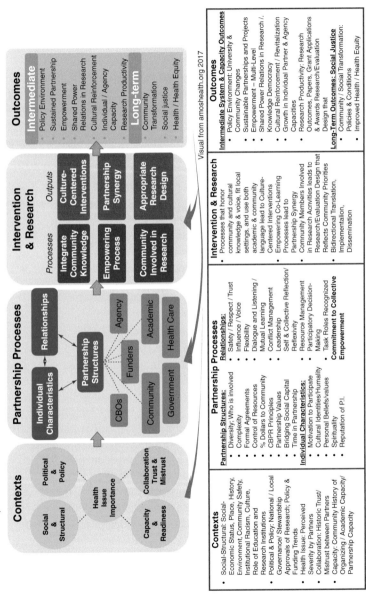

Fig. 7.3 CBPR Conceptual Model. (Adapted from Wallerstein et al. (2008) and Wallerstein and Duran (2010). Source: https://cpr.unm.edu/research-projects/cbpr-project/cbpr-model.html)

These four components within this model offer a supportive framework for designing, implementing, and evaluating CBPR health promotion projects within communities.

7.4 Assimilating Population-Focused Integrative Health Interventions to Optimize Wellness

Population-focused integrative health program management demands a focus on systems. System-oriented strategic national policies in recent decades have redirected health programs to move away from episodic-focused acute care strategies toward upstream interventions of health promotion and prevention to address root causes of health issues. These national policies and programs, including both Healthy People 2020 and 2030 plans, have expanded and specified goals to achieve optimal healthcare and wellness in the United States.

The evidence and science-based Healthy People 2020 plan is currently transitioning to Healthy People 2030, with national objectives designed to improve the health of all Americans (Healthy People 2020b). Over the past three decades, strategic national benchmarks and goals have strived to support the advancement of health promotion in the United States. The five overarching goals of the Healthy People 2030 Framework (Healthy People 2020c) target population health interventions including:

1. Attain healthy, thriving lives and well-being, free of preventable disease, disability, injury, and premature death.
2. Eliminate health disparities, achieve health equity, and attain health literacy to improve the health and well-being of all.
3. Create social, physical, and economic environments that promote attaining full potential for health and well-being for all.
4. Promote healthy development, healthy behaviors, and well-being across all life stages.
5. Engage leadership, key constituents, and the public across multiple sectors to take action and design policies that improve the health and well-being of all.

These national goals provide crucial and creative opportunities for integrative health promotion activities. Integrative health practitioners can frame community and population-focused strategies to extend interventions with specific aims within these goals. We will look at a few examples aimed toward these goals based on the integrative health equity framework.

7.4.1 An Integrative Health Equity Framework

How can integrative health services address these determinants of health to achieve health equity for optimized wellness across all populations? Trinh-Shevrin et al. (2015) proposed a promising integrative health equity framework with six main approaches and models: (1) SDOH; (2) life-course perspective; (3) CBPR approach; (4) social marketing; (5) health in all policies; and (6) bridging clinical practice and community-based health promotion.

Some significant areas to stimulate the assimilation of integrative health to optimize population-focused wellness include strengthening community-based health education and teaching strategies and programs; health advocacy and coaching models for health promotion; and the expansion of community-academic partnerships for integrative health educational programs. Community-based health education programs could be enhanced through the assimilation of integrative health interventions in such current issues as smoking cessation and vaping. Integrative health advocacy and coaching models to enhance health promotion could embrace partnering with community health worker programs and seeking policy development opportunities that target integrative health issues at county, state, and national levels.

Finally, why should we implement community-academic partnerships with integrative health educational programs? Community-academic partnerships present opportunities for students in higher educational programs, such as integrative health programs, to access community populations where students can learn to optimize the health and wellness in communities. In recent years, community-academic partnerships have emerged to bridge the growing gap in preventive health assessment and services due to public health funding cuts and other variables. These partnerships offer strategic and sustainable pathways for healthcare educational programs to assess and address the authentic community health needs and issues through focused and sustainable community engagement. These population-focused partnerships could seek to infuse integrative health interventions and approaches in community settings such as food banks; meal preparation programs; integrative health clinics and outreach centers; stress management programs at housing sites; nutrition programs, such as Nature as Pharmacy programs; state and county health department educational programs and policy development initiatives; and employee health prevention and health promotion programs with businesses, recreation centers, or fitness programs.

7.4.2   Challenges in Population-Focused Integrative Health Promotion

These opportunities for the expansion of integrative health interventions in population-focused settings to optimize wellness will require intentionality, perseverance, and strategic plans to achieve innovative integrative health programs. Some potential challenges may include sharing turf and negotiating political landscapes through interprofessional community-based partnerships; addressing quality and safety issues by advancing integrative health policies for funding and practice regulation; measuring integrative healthcare patient outcomes, particularly with a health promotion and wellness lens; and training integrative healthcare professionals to embrace population-focused integrative health initiatives and programs in communities. Despite over 20 years of moving toward a population-focused practice model, the nursing profession, specifically public health nurses, continue to face barriers to implement this innovative model to address health disparities in their own practice (Storey-Kuyl et al. 2015). Public health nurses "required significant training and support in population-focused competency development …in moving to a more complex, multilevel practice" (Espina et al. 2016). They learned key recommendations to emphasize during this training included stressing how and why population-focused practice impacts more people and how it complements rather than negates individual-level practice. Concrete examples connecting population-focused theory with individual, relationship-level and community practice strategies help to convince potential adopters of new practice models. These lessons learned by public health nurses can help to support the advancement of integrative health interventions into community settings to optimize wellness.

References

Anderson ET, McFarlane J (2011) Community as partner: theory and practice in nursing, 6th edn. Wolters Kluwer Health/Lippincott Williams & Wilkins, Philadelphia

Andrews JO, Bentley G, Crawaford S, Pretlow L, Tingen MS (2007) Using community-based participatory research to develop a culturally sensitive smoking cessation intervention with public housing neighborhoods. Ethn Dis 17(2):331–337

Centers for Disease Control and Prevention (CDC) (2019) The social ecological model: a framework for prevention model. https://www.cdc.gov/violenceprevention/publichealthissue/social-ecologicalmodel.html. Accessed 26 Nov 2019

Espina C, Bekemeier B, Storey-Kuyl M (2016) Population-focused practice competency needs among public health nursing leaders in Washington state. J Contin Educ Nurs 47(5):212–219

Hassouneh D, Alcala-Moss A, McNeff E (2011) Practical strategies for promoting full inclusion of individuals with disabilities in community-based participatory intervention research. Res Nurs Health 34:253–265

Healthy People (2020a) Social determinants of health. https://www.healthypeople.gov/2020/topics-objectives/topic/social-determinants-of-health. Accessed 26 Nov 2019

Healthy People (2020b) Educational and community-based programs. https://www.healthypeople.gov/2020/topics-objectives/topic/educational-and-community-based-programs. Accessed 26 Nov 2019

Healthly People (2020c) Healthy People 2030 framework: Overarching goals. https://www.healthypeople.gov/2020/About-Healthy-People/Development-Healthy-People-2030/Framework. Accessed 2 Dec 2020

Institute for Work and Health (2017) What researchers mean by easy to understand definitions of common research terms in the health and social sciences. https://www.iwh.on.ca/sites/iwh/files/iwh/tools/what_researchers_mean_by_2017.pdf. Accessed 21 Nov 2019

Institute of Medicine (2002) Disparities in health care methods for studying the effects of race, ethnicity and SES on access, use, and quality of health care. In: Unequal treatment confronting racial and ethnic disparities in healthcare. The National Academies Press, Washington, DC

Institute of Medicine (2003a) The future of the public's health in the twenty-first century. The National Academies Press, Washington, DC

Institute of Medicine (2003b) Who will keep the public healthy? Educating public health professionals for the 21st century. The National Academies Press, Washington, DC

Kindig D, Stoddart G (2003) What is population health? Am J Public Health 93(3):380–383

Kok G, Gottlieb NH, Commers M, Smerecnik C (2008) The ecological approach to health promotions: a decade later. Am J Health Promot 22(6):437–442

Kristjansson AL, Sigfusdottir ID, Allegrante JP, Helgason AR (2009) Parental divorce and adolescent cigarette smoking and alcohol use: assessing the importance of family conflict. Acta Paediatr 98(3):537–542

Kristjansson AL, Sigfusdottir ID, Thorlindsson T, Mann MJ, Sigfusson J, Allegrante JP (2016) Population trends in smoking, alcohol use and primary prevention variables among adolescents in Iceland, 1997–2014. Addiction 111(4):645–652

Kulbok PA, Thatcher E, Park E, Meszaros PS (2015) Evolving public health nursing roles: focus on community participatory health promotion and prevention. Online J Issues Nurs 17(2):1

Mayer K, Braband B, Killen T (2017) Exploring collaboration in a community-academic partnership. Public Health Nurs 34:541–546

Nordic Welfare Center (2019) What's new about drinking in the Nordic countries? A report on Nordic studies of adolescent drinking habits in 2000–2018. https://nordicwelfare.org/wp-content/uploads/2019/03/What%E2%80%99s-new-about-adolescent-drinking-in-the-Nordic-countries_FINAL.pdf. Accessed 14 Nov 2019

Perry C, Hoffman B (2010) Assessing tribal youth physical activity and programming using a community-based participatory research approach. Public Health Nurs 27(2):104–114

Quad Council of Public Health Nursing Organizations (2011) Care competencies for public health nurses. Quad Council of Public Health Nursing Organizations, Washington, DC

Racher FE, Annis RC (2008) Community health action model: health promotion by the community. Res Theory Nurs Pract 22(3):182–191

Sandoval JA, Lucero J, Oetzel J, Avila M, Belone L, Mau M, Pearson C, Tafoya G, Duran B, Rios LI, Wallerstein N (2012) Process and outcome constructs for evaluating community-based participatory research projects: a matrix of existing measures. Health Educ Res 27(4):680–690

Savage C, Kub J, Groves S (2016) Public health science and nursing practice: caring for populations. F.A. Davis, Philadelphia, PA

Storey-Kuyl M, Bekemeier B, Conley E (2015) Focusing "upstream" to address maternal and child inequities: two local health departments in Washington State make the transition. Matern Child Health J 19:2329–2935

Trinh-Shevrin C, Islam NS, Nadkarni S, Park R, Kwon SC (2015) Defining an integrative approach for health promotion and disease prevention: a population health equity framework. J Health Care Poor Underserved 26:146–163

U.S. Department of Health and Human Services (n.d.) Health People 2030: Framework. https://www.healthypeople.gov/2020/About-Healthy-People/Development-Healthy-People-2030/Framework. Accessed 26 Nov 2019

Wallerstein N, Duran B (2010) Community-based participatory research contributions to intervention research: the intersection of science and practice to improve health equity. Am J Public Health 100(Supp 1):540–546

Wallerstein N, Oetzel JG, Duran B et al (2008) What predicts outcomes? In: Minkler M, Wallerstein N (eds) Communication based participatory research, 2nd edn. Wiley, San Francisco

Wit CM, Chiaramonte D, Berman S, Chesney MA, Kaplan GA, Stange KC, Woolf SH, Berman BM (2017) Defining health in a comprehensive context: a new definition of integrative health. Am J Prev Med 53(1):134–137

World Health Organization (1998) Health promotion glossary. https://www.who.int/healthpromotion/HPG/en/. Accessed 14 Nov 2019

Understanding Healthcare for the Transgender and Gender Non-Confirming Community

8

Erin Waters

8.1 Introduction

To understand the needs of the transgender community, this chapter will cover information related to language, behaviors, and best practices for affirming the transgender, gender diverse, and gender non-confirming (TGN) patient population. As we continue the discussion of integrated health approaches to serving marginalized communities, overcoming challenges faced by the population must account for factors affecting including mental health, emotional stability, and ability to function within community as critical parts of the healing process. Authentic patient and practitioner partnerships are grounded in an understanding of how significantly social determinants of health influence the lives of transgender individuals, particularly those sitting at the crossroads of multiple marginalizing identity components. For a better understanding of how to work with the TGN community, it is important to understand common terms and usage.

8.1.1 Glossary

Not all transgender individuals will use the same terminology, regarding their genitals or intimate parts. Advising patients of when you will need to use specific medical terminology is helpful in alleviating concerns about identity being invalidated. Below is a condensed list of common terms used in relation to the LGBTQ+ community.

E. Waters (✉)
Equity, Inclusion and Diversity Consultant (NW), Washington, DC, USA
e-mail: Erin.Waters@kp.org

© Springer Nature Switzerland AG 2021
A. Vermeesch (ed.), *Integrative Health Nursing Interventions for Vulnerable Populations*, https://doi.org/10.1007/978-3-030-60043-3_8

8.2 Definitions (Human Rights Campaign 2019; Taylor et al. 2007; University of California, Davis 2019)

– AFAB and AMAB: Acronyms meaning "assigned female/male at birth" (also designated female/male at birth or female/male assigned at birth). No one, whether cis or trans, gets to choose what sex they're assigned at birth. This term is preferred to "biological male/female," "male/female bodied," "natal male/female," and "born male/female," which can feel deeply inaccurate.

– Gender-Affirming Surgery; Genital Reassignment/Reconstruction Surgery; Vaginoplasty; Phalloplasty; Metoidioplasty: Refers to surgical alteration, and is only one part of some trans people's transition (see "Transition" above). Only the minority of transgender people choose to and can afford to have genital surgery. The following terms are inaccurate, offensive, or outdated: sex change operation, gender reassignment/realignment surgery (gender is not changed due to surgery), gender confirmation/confirming surgery (genitalia do not confirm gender), and sex reassignment/realignment surgery (as it insinuates a single surgery is required to transition along with sex being an ambiguous term).

– Gender Binary: A system of viewing gender as consisting solely of two, opposite categories, termed "male and female," in which no other possibilities for gender or anatomy are believed to exist. This system is oppressive to anyone who defies their sex assigned at birth, but particularly those who are gender variant or do not fit neatly into one of the two standard categories.

– Passing/blending/assimilating/stealth: Being perceived by others as a particular identity/gender or cisgender regardless how the individual in question identifies, e.g., passing as straight, passing as a cis woman, passing as a youth. This term has become controversial as "passing" can imply that one is not genuinely what they are passing as. (Note, to be "clocked" is to be identified as transgender without intentional revealing, aka the opposite of the words being defined here).

– Sexual orientation.

    An inherent or immutable enduring emotional, romantic, or sexual attraction to other people.

– Gender identity.

    One's innermost concept of self as male, female, a blend of both or neither—how individuals perceive themselves and what they call themselves. One's gender identity can be the same or different from their sex assigned at birth.

– Gender expression.

    External appearance of one's gender identity, usually expressed through behavior, clothing, haircut, or voice, and which may or may not conform to socially defined behaviors and characteristics typically associated with being either masculine or feminine.

– Transgender.

    An umbrella term for people whose gender identity and/or expression is different from cultural expectations based on the sex they were assigned at birth. Being transgender does not imply any specific sexual orientation. Therefore, transgender people may identify as straight, gay, lesbian, bisexual, etc.

- Gender transition.

  The process by which some people strive to more closely align their internal knowledge of gender with its outward appearance. Some people socially transition, whereby they might begin dressing, using names and pronouns and/or be socially recognized as another gender. Others undergo physical transitions in which they modify their bodies through medical interventions. Read more.
- Gender dysphoria.

  Clinically significant distress caused when a person's assigned birth gender is not the same as the one with which they identify. According to the American Psychiatric Association's Diagnostic and Statistical Manual of Mental Disorders (DSM), the term—which replaces Gender Identity Disorder—"is intended to better characterize the experiences of affected children, adolescents, and adults."

8.2.1   Identities

- Cisgender: a gender identity, or performance in a gender role, that society deems to match the person's assigned sex at birth. The prefix cis- means "on this side of" or "not across." A term used to call attention to the privilege of people who are not transgender.
- Culture: A learned set of values, beliefs, customs, norms, and perceptions shared by a group of people that provide a general design for living and a pattern for interpreting life. "Culture is those deep, common, unstated, learned experiences which members of a given culture share, which they communicate without knowing, and which form the backdrop against which all other events are judged."
- Gender: A social construct used to classify a person as a man, woman, or some other identity. Fundamentally different from the sex one is assigned at birth. Gender can be considered as one's internal sense of being a man, woman, both, neither, or something else. Whereas many individuals feel alignment in terms of the sex they were assigned at birth and their gender are cisgender (cis; Latin. "same") as a result, some individuals do not have similar alignment and may identify as transgender (trans; latin. "across"). Individuals who identify outside of expected or assumed binary interpretations of gender identity (re: male/female) may see themselves as non-binary or identified.
- Gender Expansive: An umbrella term used for individuals who broaden their own culture's commonly held definitions of gender, including expectations for its expression, identities, roles, and/or other perceived gender norms. Gender expansive individuals include those who identify as transgender, as well as anyone else whose gender in some way is seen to be stretching the surrounding society's notion of gender.
- Gender Fluid: A person whose gender identification and presentation shifts, whether within or outside of societal, gender-based expectations. Being fluid in motion between two or more genders.

- Gender Identity: A sense of one's self as trans*, genderqueer, woman, man, or some other identity, which may or may not correspond with the sex and gender one is assigned at birth.
- Gender Non-conforming (GNC): people who do not subscribe to gender expressions or roles expected of them by society.
- Gender roles reflect attitudes and expectations a given culture associates with certain sexes/genders. Behavior which conforms to those expectations can be called gender-conforming or gender-normative; behavior that does not meet those expectations can be considered gender non-conforming or gender-nonnormative.
- Gender Queer: A person whose gender identity and/or gender expression falls outside of the dominant societal norm for their assigned sex, is beyond genders, or is some combination of them.
- Heteronormativity: A set of lifestyle norms, practices, and institutions that promote binary alignment of biological sex, gender identity, and gender roles; assume heterosexuality as a fundamental and natural norm; and privilege monogamous, committed relationships and reproductive sex above all other sexual practices.
- Heterosexism: The assumption that all people are or should be heterosexual. Heterosexism excludes the needs, concerns, and life experiences of lesbian, gay, bisexual, and queer people while it gives advantages to heterosexual people. It is often a subtle form of oppression, which reinforces realities of silence and erasure.
- Heterosexuality: A sexual orientation in which a person feels physically and emotionally attracted to people of a gender other than their own.
- Homosexual/Homosexuality: A term to describe a sexual orientation in which a person feels physically and emotionally attracted to people of the same gender.
- Intersex: Adjective used to describe the experience of naturally (that is, without any medical intervention) developing primary or secondary sex characteristics that do not fit neatly into society's definitions of male or female. Intersex is an umbrella term and there are around 20 variations of intersex that are included in this umbrella term. Many visibly intersex people are subjected to genital surgery during infancy and early childhood by doctors to make the individual's sex characteristics conform to society's idea of what [binary] bodies should look like. Intersex people are relatively common, although society…has allowed very little room for intersex issues to be discussed publicly. It is important to note that intersex and transgender are different terms and not all transgender individuals are intersex, nor do all intersex individuals identify as transgender.
- Lesbian: A woman whose primary sexual and affectional orientation is toward people of the same gender.
- LGBT: Abbreviation for Lesbian, Gay, Bisexual, and Transgender. An umbrella term that is often used to refer to the community as a whole. Our center uses LGBTQIA to intentionally include and raise awareness of Queer, Intersex and Asexual as well as myriad of other communities under our umbrella.

- Misgendering: Attributing a gender to someone that is incorrect/does not align with their gender identity. Can occur when using pronouns, gendered language (i.e., "Hello ladies!" "Hey guys"), or assigning genders to people without knowing how they identify (i.e., "Well, since we're all women in this room, we understand…").
- Non-binary: A gender identity and experience that embraces a full universe of expressions and ways of being that resonate for an individual. It may be an active resistance to binary gender expectations and/or an intentional creation of new unbounded ideas of self within the world. For some people who identify as non-binary, there may be overlap with other concepts and identities like gender expansive and gender non-conforming.
- Orientation: Orientation is one's attraction or non-attraction to other people. An individual's orientation can be fluid and people use a variety of labels to describe their orientation. Some, but not all, types of attraction or orientation include: romantic, sexual, sensual, aesthetic, intellectual, and platonic.
- Pronouns: Linguistic tools used to refer to someone in the third person. Examples are they/them/theirs, ze/hir/hirs, she/her/hers, he/him/his. In English and some other languages, pronouns have been tied to gender and are a common site of misgendering (attributing a gender to someone that is incorrect). In terms of pronouns, many use she/her or he/him pronouns as one would expect in a binary understanding of gender (e.g., "he went to the store," "she is sitting in that chair"). Non-binary or gender-fluid identified individuals may use they/them pronouns (they went to the store, I want to talk with them). It can take some adjustment to adjust pronouns, particularly with unfamiliar pronouns (e.g., xe/xir, zey/zir). In those moments, use of a proper noun or an individual's name is best practice.
- Queer: One definition of queer is abnormal or strange. Historically, queer has been used as an epithet/slur against people whose gender, gender expression, and/or sexuality do not conform to dominant expectations. Some people have reclaimed the word queer and self-identify as such. For some, this reclamation is a celebration of not fitting into norms/being "abnormal." Manifestations of oppression within gay and lesbian movements such as racism, sizeism, ableism, cissexism, transmisogyny as well as assimilation politics, resulted in many people being marginalized, thus, for some, queer is a radical and anti-assimilationist stance that captures multiple aspects of identities. Historically queer was used as a slur but has been reclaimed and adopted by some members of the community. In general, this identity marker is used to signify someone who does not want traditional expectations about their gender or sexual orientation to be applied. It is important to allow individuals to provide this as their identity marker as making assumptions may result in assumed negative intent.
- Sex: a medically constructed categorization. Sex is often assigned based on the appearance of the genitalia, either in ultrasound or at birth. Sex is currently classified as male, female, or intersex. Regarding the transgender community, sex can be considered "assigned" as birth and is generally based on external genitalia. It is important to note that transgender and intersex are different and have

differing medical implications; individuals who are transgender are not necessarily intersex and vice versa.

- Sexual Orientation: Sexual Orientation is an enduring emotional, romantic, sexual, or affectional attraction or non-attraction to other people. Sexual orientation can be fluid and people use a variety of labels to describe their sexual orientation.
- Transgender: Adjective used most often as an umbrella term and frequently abbreviated to "trans." This adjective describes a wide range of identities and experiences of people whose gender identity and/or expression differs from conventional expectations based on their assigned sex at birth. Not all trans people undergo medical transition (surgery or hormones). Some commonly held definitions:

  Someone whose determination of their sex and/or gender is not validated by dominant societal expectations; someone whose behavior or expression does not "match" their assigned sex according to society.
  A gender outside of the man/woman binary.
  Having no gender or multiple genders.

- Transition: An individualized process by which transsexual and transgender people "switch" from one gender presentation to another. There are three general aspects to transitioning: social (i.e., name, pronouns, interactions, etc.), medical (i.e., hormones, surgery, etc.), and legal (i.e., gender marker, name change, etc.). A trans individual may transition in any combination, or none, of these aspects. In some cases, transgender individuals may wish for medical intervention to accompany transition. Transition is a period or process in which individuals may make social, legal, physical, or other changes to affirming their identity. For the largest majority of transgender individuals, transition is the most effective method of treatment with the highest outcomes (Bränström 2019). Rates of regret and detransition remain exceedingly low (Danker et al. 2018), with primary reasoning being social, romantic, and familial rejection. However, not all transgender and gender non-conforming (TGN) individuals seek medical intervention in relation to their identity or as part of their transition process. It is important to allow an individual to identify their own pathway and then provide them avenues of access and support to meeting those transition-related goals.
- Two Spirit: "[This] term stems from the Ojibwe phrase niizh manidoowag and replaces the outdated, oversimplified term berdache, which appeared frequently in research and anthropological studies that aimed to describe the place of gay men in Native society in the eighteenth and early nineteenth centuries [...] The phrase 'two spirit' began to gain traction across Native America after 1990, when 13 men, women, and transgender people from various tribes met in Winnipeg, Canada, with the task of finding a term that could unite the LGBTQ Native community. [...] For me, the term 'two spirit' resists a Western definition of who we are and what we should be. Two spirit [people] are integral to the struggle of undoing the impacts of historical trauma, because our roles in tribes historically were part of the traditions taken away from us with Westernization."—Zachary

Pullin (Chippewa Cree), May/June 2014 Issues of Native Peoples (Note: There are a variety of definitions and feelings about the term "two spirit"—and this term does not resonate for everyone.) The term "Two Spirit" is also used by some individuals in Indigenous and Native communities for those who are transgender, non-binary, or otherwise gender non-conforming (Taylor 2009).

8.3   Gender Equity

As time proceeds we are seeing a cultural shift toward gender and equity. This is particularly noteworthy in terms of the medical community's expanding support for transgender, gender diverse, and gender non-conforming individuals (TGN). Healthcare coverage providers and insurers are increasingly offering covered benefits for transition-related care, resulting in increased access to care. Improved access means more providers are encountering TGN individuals and need for better ways of providing competent care grows. Disrupting and dispelling bias is critical first step in the equal provision of adequate care to all patient populations. Providers are asked not only to treat the patient, but to inquire about a larger picture to better understand the individuals and unique challenges faced by a patient outside of the exam room. Undertaking the effort to ensure one is aware of current evidence in support, leading best practices, and history of the TGN community's continual fight for equity moves providers beyond seeing patients as a list of diagnoses. Instead, they relate holistically to a whole person with a collection of lived experiences.

Research shows that affirming the identities of TGN patients significantly improves overall healthcare outcomes (Russell et al. 2018; Sevelius 2013). In addition, the largest majority of health professional organizations have stated affirmation and support of TNG patients in their identities leads to the best outcomes and engagement (Legal 2018). "Conversion therapy" or "reparative therapy" refers to practices aimed at changing an individual's sexual orientation or gender identity. Like with the larger LGBQ+ population, conversion therapy is not only ineffective, but actively harmful to both short- and long-term stability in healthcare outcomes (Toomey and Anhalt 2016). In some cases, practice conversion therapy is illegal, especially regarding TGN youth (American Psychiatric Association Board of Trustees 2018; Toomey and Anhalt 2016).

Unfortunately, due to historical and structural issues related to healthcare systems and practices, the community struggles with significant distrust in healthcare providers. Much of the current healthcare aversion experienced by the patient population is due to provider discrimination (Grant et al. 2011; James et al. 2016), followed by a lack of provider knowledge (Grant et al. 2011). Healthcare aversion can be reduced most noticeably through affirmation of identity, followed by motivational interviewing techniques, and using trauma-informed care principles (Toomey and Anhalt 2016).

In addition to general difficulties, the population faces in finding competent providers willing to give care, issues related to compounding identities can exacerbate existing community challenges. Factors such as socioeconomic status can be compounded with other demographic other factors, such as race or sexual orientation resulting in intersections of various identities (Williams-Crenshaw 1994). As these identities compound, systemic barriers increase and outcomes further decline. When aggregating data, the introduction of variables such as race, socioeconomic status, and LGBTQIA2S+ identity consistently result in worsening outcomes. The combination of anti-transgender bias and persistent, structural racism in particular can be especially devastating; Black, Indigenous, and people of color in general fare worse than white counterparts across the board, with African American transgender respondents having least positive outcomes in most areas in which disparity is examined (Taylor 2009).

There is a tendency to assume being transgender is a unique or new in the course of human history (Restar 2018). However, there is proof of gender variant, diverse, and non-conforming people through history, often identified in ancient cultures such as the Hijra in India and two-spirit identities (Mesa-Miles 2014; Pullin 2014; Turban et al. 2019), a term used to describe gender-variant individuals in indigenous communities across the Americas.

More modern history is seen in the 1930s Germany where the Institute for Sex Research (Institut für Sexualwissenschaft) studied and treated transgender individuals in affirmation of their identities. With the rise of Nazism in Germany, the institute was burned to the ground destroying the largest body of peer-reviewed medical research on transgender individuals (Grau and Schoppmann 1995).

In 1980, the American Psychiatric Association classified transgender individuals as having "gender identity disorder" (Stryker 2004). This was followed by increased engagement from medical professionals in discussing the phenomenon of transgender individuals. There was resulting backlash from the lesbian community, prompting transgender author Sandy Stone to write the essay "The Empire Strikes Back: A Posttranssexual Manifesto" (Stone 1987). However, the United States' Health & Human Services Department clarified that Medicare did not cover gender-affirming surgeries (Trans Student Educational Resources 2019).

In 2012, the American Psychiatric Association's board of trustees approved changes to The Diagnostic and Statistical Manual of Mental Disorders (DSM-V). It removed the term "Gender Identity Disorder" (GID) as a mental health diagnosis. The term "Gender Dysphoria" became the standard used to describe emotional distress over "a marked incongruence between one's experienced/expressed gender and assigned gender."

In some cases, the law has evolved to help reduce discrimination against TGN Americans. Section 1557 of the Affordable Care Act prohibits entities that receive federal funding for health coverage from denying coverage based on sex, gender identity, and sex stereotyping (United States Center for Medicaid and Services 1989). The Americans with Disabilities Act and Title VII of the Civil Rights Act have also been broadly interpreted by courts to protect transgender individuals from discrimination.

8.3.1 Social Determinants of Health (SDOH)

To understand some of the complexities in the lives of transgender individuals, it is important to reflect on how additionally difficult being TGN can be in cultures still learning how to be affirming and creating space for these identities.

Social determinants of health are conditions in the environments in which people are born, live, learn, work, play, worship, and age that affect a wide range of health, functioning, and quality-of-life outcomes and risks. Conditions (e.g., social, economic, and physical) in these various environments and settings (e.g., school, church, workplace, and neighborhood) affect patterns of social engagement, sense of security, and overall well-being. Resources that enhance quality of life can have a significant influence on population health outcomes. Examples of these resources include safe and affordable housing, access to education, public safety, availability of healthy foods, local emergency/health services, and environments free of life-threatening toxins (United States Department of Health and Human Services Department 2016).

It is fundamentally important to remember that understanding how various identity-markers a person holds can overlap, creating significantly worse outcomes and access to resources (Williams-Crenshaw 1994). A person who is transgender may experience significant difficulty in accessing affirming, resources, or affirming care. But, if they also embody other identities such as Black, Indigenous, or being a person of color (BIPOC), disabled, being a senior, or large-bodied/fat those difficulties can exponentially increase. These increases are the result of both small and large biases, both conscious and unconscious, inherent in individuals and systems built with little consideration for how these identities intertwine to create unique challenges for marginalized identities. Examples within the transgender community include (Grant et al. 2011; James et al. 2016; Virupaksha et al. 2016):

- 29% of transgender people live in poverty, compared to 14% of the general population.
- 30% of transgender people report being homeless at some point in their lives, with 12% saying it was within the past 12 months.
- Transgender people experience unemployment at 3× the rate of the general population, with rates for people of color up to 4× the national unemployment rate.
- 30% of transgender people report being fired, denied a promotion, or experiencing mistreatment in the workplace due to their gender identity in the past 12 months.
- 31% of transgender people experienced mistreatment in the past year in a place of public accommodation, including 14% who were denied equal service, 24% who were verbally harassed, and 2% who were physically attacked because they were transgender.
- 40% of respondents reported attempting suicide in their lifetime, nearly nine times the attempted suicide rate in the United States (4.6%).

A clear understanding of the term "intersectionality" can be helpful in approaching an integrated and comprehensive view of patient care. Intersectionality is a term coined by law professor Kimberlé Crenshaw in the 1980s to describe the way that multiple systems of oppression interact in the lives of those with multiple marginalized identities. Intersectionality looks at the relationships between multiple marginalized identities and allows us to analyze social problems more fully, shape more effective interventions, and promote more inclusive advocacy amongst communities.

Individuals with backgrounds in social work and trauma-informed care principles can help identify community resources that are both affirming and supportive of TGN identities. Trust development in this context is challenging, as referral to community organizations which are not supportive of TGN individuals will erode trust and play into a larger narrative of healthcare aversion due. For example, a food pantry may be associated with an organization whose values run counter to supporting the TGN community. Accurate identification of resources that are affirming in addition to consistently steering patent away from those which are not is foundational in building trust with members of the community. Lack of consistent professional support means individuals rely heavily on each other and word of mouth to transfer information related to safety in approaching affirming providers.

To reduce disparities, health and community systems are increasingly developing avenues for engagement with community health workers. Some states have formal networks of community health workers while many others represent motivated individuals. The differences between non-licensed community health workers and licensed social workers revolve heavily around clinical assessment and ability to provide acute mental health support (Spencer et al. 2010).

8.3.2 Barriers to Care

There are a variety of barriers to accessing care; however, it primarily revolves around lack of general access and lack of understanding how to treat the population. In addition to SDOH, the most significant barrier to accessing care is lack of cultural humility/competency in terms of provider knowledge, which may often be paired with unconscious bias, implicit bias, and active discrimination (Grant et al. 2011). Despite increased support for LGBTQ+ identities, widespread discrimination persists (Herek and McLemore 2013).

There are significant SDOH factors in play when it comes to occupying TGN identities. Gender-based victimization, discrimination, bullying, violence, being rejected by the family, friends, and community; harassment by intimate partner, family members, police, and public; discrimination and ill-treatment at healthcare systems are significant factors. These issues contribute to difficulty navigating the word at large, with ill-treatment at healthcare systems being a significant factor. In all cases, these issues and fears related to them contribute to increased rates of suicidality within the TGN community (Toomey and Anhalt 2016; United States Department of Health and Human Services Department 2016).

Many TGN individuals have difficult or even discriminatory experiences with the medical system. A survey of transgender adolescents and adults from Ontario, Canada found that more than half of respondents reported a negative experience during care in an emergency department, and at least 1 in 5 had avoided the emergency room due to fears that their gender identity may negatively affect their care (Guss et al. 2015). The National Transgender Discrimination Survey, a national retrospective survey study of TGN adults in the USA, found that half of respondents postponed seeking medical care when they were sick due to discrimination or financial concerns (James et al. 2016).

Discrimination can also be found in the form of minimizing issues dealing with gender dysphoria. While there are studies claiming that gender dysphoria can onset rapidly or that the increased prevalence of those identifying as transgender have increased (Restar 2018), these studies primarily represent a repackaging of the social contagion theory (Christakisa 2013; Knauer 2000). The primary difference between TGN individuals now and throughout history is that more cultures are making room for increased gender variance and exploration. Such as the case with the gay and lesbian community, the social contagion theory outlines the idea that peer pressure is what drives individuals to identify as LGBTQ+ in some way. Working from a contagion model, being transgender is framed as an immoral, unhealthy, and/or freely chosen vice. However, position statements from leading medical organizations dispute this idea and agree that affirmation of identity is the best method producing positive outcomes for the population (Legal 2018).

Historically, information related to the care and support of the transgender community has gone overlooked in healthcare settings (Obedin-Maliver et al. 2011). This lack of knowledge can lead to reluctance in care provision in addition to lack of competent provision when required. Approximately one in ten transgender individuals experience a reduction in quality of care once a provider identifies them as TGN (Grant et al. 2011). Lack of medical provider knowledge can make patients feel unwelcome and can hinder appropriate referral for mental health or hormonal interventions. A survey of medical schools in 2009–2010 found that the median number of hours of LGBT content was 5 hours with one-third of schools reporting no LGBT curriculum during the clinical years (Obedin-Maliver et al. 2011). Additionally, in a medical school class in Philadelphia, 74% of respondents had 2 hours or less of transgender health topics in medical school. However, the Philadelphia students who received an additional lecture on transgender health during their clerkship years had improved knowledge, attitudes, and skills compared to students who had not received the lecture (Obedin-Maliver et al. 2011). Thus, the addition of even one lecture in medical school may improve provider competency in caring for TGN patients.

Insurance coverage represents an additional barrier to care for TGN patients. In the USA, cross-hormone or pubertal suppressive therapies are prescribed off-label and may be denied by insurance companies. Gender-affirming surgery is not consistently covered by insurance and is cost-prohibitive for many outside of medical insurance provision. Broad exclusions, narrow inclusions, and limited lifetime amounts on what patients can use toward transition-related care can leave many in the difficult position of having to choose an incomplete transition path. However, progress is being made in this arena. At the time of this publication, multiple US states have Medicaid programs that explicitly cover medical services for the treatment of gender dysphoria (Mallory 2019). It is reasonable to expect that this trend toward increased inclusivity will continue in all levels of insurance provision.

8.4   Important Areas of Consideration

There are common areas of engagement and therefore important areas of consideration when working with the TGN community. Bathroom avoidance is a problem. Consistent with typical hormone therapy protocols used for transgender women, anti-androgens such as spironolactone and finasteride (Deutsch 2016) are diuretics which can increase need for bathroom usage. From the 2015 US Trans Survey (James et al. 2016), the following areas for consideration were identified:

- 59% of respondents reported that in the past year they had either sometimes (48%) or always (11%) avoided using a restroom, such as in public, at work, or at school, because they were afraid of confrontations or other problems.
- 12% report that they have been harassed, attacked, or sexually assaulted in a bathroom in the last year.
- Transgender men (75%) were far more likely to report sometimes or always avoiding using a public restroom, in contrast to transgender women (53%) and non-binary respondents (53%).
- Undocumented residents were also more likely to report sometimes or always avoiding using a public restroom in the past year (72%).
- Eighty percent (80%) of respondents who said that others could always or usually tell that they were transgender and 72% of those who said that others can sometimes tell they are transgender reported avoiding using public restroom, in contrast to 48% of those who said that others can rarely or never tell that they are transgender.
- 31% have avoided drinking or eating so that they did not need to use the restroom in the last year.
- 24% report that someone told them they were using the wrong restroom or questioned their presence in the restroom in the last year.
- 9% report being denied access to the appropriate restroom in the last year.
- These issues above resulted in 8% reporting having a kidney or urinary tract infection, or another kidney-related medical issue, from avoiding restrooms in the last year.

There is increased prevalence in eating disorders within the transgender community, though the occurrence is higher in AFAB individuals over AMAB individuals. Results in a 2018 study of 452 adult transgender patients (Diemer et al. 2018) identified the age-adjusted odds of self-reported ED in MTF participants were 0.14 times the odds of self-reported ED in FBGNC participants ($p = 0.022$). In FTM participants, the age-adjusted odds of self-reported ED were 0.46 times the odds of self-reported ED in FBGNC participants, a marginally significant finding ($p = 0.068$).

The crux of the issue is a lack of control over the body and changes associated with a puberty inconsistent with the held gender identity of the individual (Diemer et al. 2018; Rood et al. 2016; Redcay 2015; Taylor 2009). Healthcare providers can improve equitable outcomes through education on possible differences regarding prevalence, age of onset, persistence, and gender differences in eating disorders to appropriately assess, and diagnose eating disorders among subgroups of minority populations (Taylor 2009).

In terms of surgery, as with any patient in emergency situations due to surgical complications, it is best to contact the patient's surgeon directly. Providers for some procedures are limited, particularly phalloplasty and vaginoplasty surgeries. Identifying who may be in your area and ensuring contact information is on file will reduce delays in identifying appropriate triage responses.

Providers who demonstrate an understanding of potential transition goals and timelines will more effectively generate trust with patients. There are a significant number of resources available to understand both recommendations (World Professional Association for Transgender Health 2019) and clinical guidelines (Deutsch 2016) related to TGN patients seeking gender-affirming medical transition. Intentionally addressing timelines is a necessary step in education to provide realistic context for noticeable changes while ensuring sound medical decision-making is being utilized by both patient and practitioner.

As an example of a common timeline for someone who begins transition early/pre-puberty:

- Prepubertal: social transition only with no medical intervention(s).
- Puberty: Administration of pubertal delaying agent (Clemons et al. 1993; Deutsch 2016; Olson-Kennedy et al. 2016).
- Age 14–15: begin cross-sex hormone replacement therapy (HRT) regimen.
- 18+: surgical intervention(s) as desired.

Guidelines set forth by the World Professional Association for Transgender Health (World Professional Association for Transgender Health 2019) require TGN individuals to receive various assessments from qualified mental health practitioners (QMHP) before accessing certain medical interventions. Adult patients are increasingly utilizing informed-consent models for HRT, whereas more specific assessments are required for surgical intervention. These assessments outline dysphoric intensity while affirming TGN patients can make sound medical decisions. Specific, youth-focused assessments must be completed for minors.

8.4.1   Common Post-Surgical Complications

- "Top" surgery (e.g., bilateral mastectomy, chest contouring; breast augmentation via saline, silicone, or autologous fat grafting): pain, infection, seroma, hematoma, some degree of wound separation, delayed wound healing, or skin flap necrosis, capsular contracture, dehiscence, symmastia, implant migration, hematoma, and potential implant extrusion/exposure (Barton et al. 2005; Wang and Kim 2016; Xu et al. 2019).

– Genital surgery (e.g., phalloplasty, metoidioplasty, vaginoplasty, vulvoplasty): hematoma, torn stitches, odor, discharge, stenosis, urethral stricture, urinary tract infection (UTI), fistula, granulation tissue, and necrotic tissue (Djordjevic et al. 2019; Dreher et al. 2018; Jun and Santucci 2019; Rashid and Sarmad-Tamimy 2013).

8.4.2 Population-Specific Methods for Stress Reduction

When we discuss stress reduction, it is important for us to acknowledge the sources of stress under which the TGN community struggle. Integrative approaches to healing TGN patients involve commitment to understanding how social determinants reduce mental and psychological safety in the population as community may be lacking due systemic or negatively biased forces outside of their control. Affirming medical care can mend historically broken relationships between the TGN community and healthcare systems, circumventing and ultimately improving areas of limited patient functionality.

Primary/Major Stressors (**Rood et al. 2016**):
– Being "outed" or identified as transgender ("clocked" is a slang term used within the community to denote being identified or recognized as transgender without having intentionally revealed oneself).
– Lack of affirmation of identity (being repeatedly and intentionally misgendered).
– Expectations of rejection.
– Lack of knowledge of the transgender community.
– Lack of empathy for the significance of gender dysphoria.

Traditional methods of stress reduction such as exercise can be challenging for TGN patients, as those who are early in transition are likely to fear being in public due to safety concerns. Encouraging meditation and self-reflection is a good alternative. Encouraging participation in social groups is also beneficial. Note that TGN patients are not guaranteed to find safety or affirmation with other members of the LGBQ+ community; be sure recommendations include referral to organization that are confirmed to be supportive of TGN identities.

8.5   Conclusion

In conclusion, best practices to help with stress reduction on the transgender community are:

1. Avoid using gendered pronouns whenever possible.
   (a) Examples include calling patients back into exam spaces or confirming identity once there.

2. Use alternate methods of verifying identity when working with trans patients.
   (a) It is common to use first name and birthdate as means of identity confirmation. However, many patients are unable to change their names due to economic concerns or in some cases legal or social issues which prevent them from doing so. In those cases, refer to the header of your electronic medical record (EMR) for additional markers that would help identify the patient.
   (b) Examples: last name, date of birth, listed telephone number, unique allergy information, etc.
   (c) Note, if the EMR you are working with does not capture SOGI information, it would be beneficial to encourage your organization to seek out relevant updates which will allow you to capture the information consistently and display it prominently.
3. Do not assume a TGN patient's pronouns based on their presentation.
   (a) In some cases, non-binary identified patients may present in ways that seem to fit into binary expectations. Other patients may not be able to dress or present in ways that would typically match cultural expectations related to specific genders.
   (b) Assuming based on appearance can result in significant errors (e.g., assumptions that a woman with a short haircut wearing jeans who identifies as lesbian must also transgender.)
4. Offer your own name and pronouns first.
   (a) This will provide an opportunity for you to get to know your patient, but also level set. If you are offering your name and pronouns with the expectation that they will be respected, it creates an environment in which a TNG person will feel more confident offering theirs and that their identity will be affirmed during encounters.
5. If you make a mistake, apologize and move forward.
   (a) A common error is to spend a significant amount of time justifying or explaining why a mistake happened. It is important to acknowledge the error, present the correct information and then affirm that will be used going forward. Time spent over-explaining and/or justifying the error will result in awkward feelings for both you and the patient. If we liken those awkward feelings to a balloon, we understand that someone during the encounter must hold it. Either you must due to feelings of guilt and concern or the patient must in which they may end up apologize the more time spent deflecting.
   (b) Most importantly, it is best not to put a patient in the position of having to apologize or reassure you if you are the one who made a mistake in affirming their identity.
      • Remember, it is the healthcare provider's job to create a space of safety and affirming for a patient. It is not a patient's job to coddle us in our errors.
6. Use a patient's correct name/pronouns even when the patient is not present.
   (a) While we may feel that we will be able to switch between present legal name and the name they actually use effectively, developing good habits early is important.

7. Encourage coworkers who are not affirming identity to do so at every opportunity.
   (a) Creating affirming environments that are inclusive of all bodies requires a collective effort from all corners.
8. Remember that SOGI information is Protected Health Information (PHI).
   (a) Giving that information out even to coworkers may inadvertently "out" a patient, which can have significant consequences in terms of housing, employment, and access to resources as a whole.
   (b) If a patient wishes to reveal this information to someone that is their choice. Beyond that we must understand that it is a violation of HIPAA to give it out without explicit permission.
9. Avoid "curiosity" questions (Knutson et al. 2016) and seek active consent.
   (a) As with any patient, we want to ensure the information we request is relevant to the presented issue. Not doing so is known as the "trans broken arm syndrome," in which a transgender patient presents with an issue such as a broken arm, but the provider asks questions related to gender-affirming surgery history which has no relevance to healthcare concern at hand.
10. Remember that patients who have intersecting identities (disabled, BIPOC, age, etc.) may experience a significantly higher number of challenges when accessing care and navigating through the larger community (Sevelius 2013).

References

American Psychiatric Association Board of Trustees (2018) Position statement on conversion therapy and LGBTQ patients. Conversion Therapy—APA statement. https://www.psychiatry.org/home/policy-finder

Barton MB, West CN, Liu IL, Harris EL, Rolnick SJ, Elmore JG et al (2005) Complications following bilateral prophylactic mastectomy. J Natl Cancer Inst Monogr 35:61–66. Complications following bilateral prophylactic mastectomy: https://www.ncbi.nlm.nih.gov/pubmed/16287887

Bränström P (2019) Reduction in mental health treatment utilization among transgender individuals after gender-affirming surgeries: a total population study. Am J Psychiatry 177:727–734. https://doi.org/10.1176/appi.ajp.2019.19010080

Christakisa F (2013) Social contagion theory: examining dynamic social networks and human behavior. Stat Med 32(4):556–577. Social Contagion Theory: https://www.ncbi.nlm.nih.gov/pmc/articles/PMC3830455/

Clemons RD, Kappy MS, Stuart TE, Perelman AH, Hoekstra FT (1993) Long-term effectiveness of depot gonadotropin-releasing hormone analogue in the treatment of children with central precocious puberty. Am J Dis Child 147(6):653–657. Lupron Efficacy: https://www.ncbi.nlm.nih.gov/pubmed/8506834

Danker S, Narayan SK, Bluebond-Langner R, Schechter LS, Berli JU (2018) A survey study of surgeons' experience with regret and/or reversal of gender-confirmation surgeries (abstract). Plast Reconstr Surg Glob Open 6(9 Suppl):189–189. Detransition: https://www.ncbi.nlm.nih.gov/pmc/articles/PMC6212091/

Deutsch (2016) Guidelines for the primary and gender-affirming care of transgender and gender nonbinary people, 2nd edn. University of California, San Francisco. https://transcare.ucsf.edu/guidelines

Diemer EW, White Hughto JM, Gordon AR, Guss C, Austin SB, Reisner SL (2018) Beyond the binary: differences in eating disorder prevalence by gender identity in a transgender sample. Transgend Health 3(1):17–23. https://www.ncbi.nlm.nih.gov/pmc/articles/PMC5775111/

Djordjevic ML, Stojanovic B, Bizic M (2019) Metoidioplasty: techniques and outcomes. Transl Androl Urol 8(3):248–253. https://www.ncbi.nlm.nih.gov/pmc/articles/PMC6626308/

Dreher PC, Edwards D, Hager S, Dennis M, Belkoff A, Mora J, Tarry S, Rumer KL (2018) Complications of the neovagina in male-to-female transgender surgery: a systematic review and meta-analysis with discussion of management. Clin Anat 31(2):191–199. https://www.ncbi.nlm.nih.gov/pubmed/29057562

Grant J, Mottet L, Tanis J, Herman JL, Harrison J, Keisling M (2011) Injustice at every turn: a report of the National Transgender Discrimination Survey. National Center for Transgender Equality and National Gay and Lesbian Task Force, Washington, DC. https://www.transequality.org/sites/default/files/docs/resources/NTDS_Report.pdf

Grau G, Schoppmann C (1995) The hidden holocaust?: Gay and Lesbian persecution in Germany 1933–45. Taylor and Francis, London

Guss C, Shumer D, Katz-Wise SL (2015) Transgender and gender nonconforming adolescent care: psychosocial and medical considerations. Curr Opin Pediatr 26(4):421–426. TGN Adolescent Care: https://www.ncbi.nlm.nih.gov/pmc/articles/PMC4522917/

Herek GM, McLemore KA (2013) Sexual prejudice. Annu Rev Psychol 64:309–333. https://doi.org/10.1146/annurev-psych-113011-143826

Human Rights Campaign (2019) Sexual orientation and gender identity definitions. https://www.hrc.org/resources/sexual-orientation-and-gender-identity-terminology-and-definitions

James SE, Herman JL, Rankin S, Keisling M, Mottet L, Anafi M (2016) The report of the 2015 U.S. transgender survey. National Center for Transgender Equality, Washington, DC. https://transequality.org/sites/default/files/docs/usts/USTS-Full-Report-Dec17.pdf

Jun MS, Santucci RA (2019) Urethral stricture after phalloplasty. Transl Androl Urol 8(3):266–272. (abstract). Urethral stricture after phalloplasty: http://tau.amegroups.com/article/view/25970/24258

Knauer NJ (2000) Homosexuality as contagion: from the well of loneliness to the boy scouts. Hofstra Law Rev 29(2):Article 2. https://scholarlycommons.law.hofstra.edu/cgi/viewcontent.cgi?article=2118&context=hlr

Knutson D, Koch JM, Arthur T, Mitchell TA, Martyr MA (2016) Trans broken arm: health care stories from transgender people in rural areas. J Res Women Gend 7:30–46. (abstract) https://pdfs.semanticscholar.org/32e4/3561a59a49c3cbc32f4e1983b52112495da2.pdf

Legal L (2018) Professional organization statements supporting transgender people in healthcare. In: Professional position statements. https://www.lambdalegal.org/publications/fs_professional-org-statements-supporting-trans-health

Mallory T (2019) Medicaid coverage for gender-affirming care. The Williams Institute. LGBT Medicaid Map, Los Angeles, CA. https://www.lgbtmap.org/img/maps/citations-medicaid.pdf

Mesa-Miles (2014) Two spirit: the trials and tribulations of gender identity in the 21st century. Indian Country Today. https://newsmaven.io/indiancountrytoday/archive/two-spirit-the-trials-and-tribulations-of-gender-identity-in-the-21st-century-vJO2nkYbLkCiOWXteDhjsw/. Accessed 11 Nov 2019

Obedin-Maliver J, Goldsmith ES, Stewart L, White W, Tran E, Brenman S, Wells M, Fetterman DM, Garcia G, Lunn MR (2011) Lesbian, gay, bisexual, and transgender-related content in undergraduate medical education. JAMA 306(9):971–977. Lesbian, gay, bisexual, and transgender-related content in undergraduate medical education. https://www.ncbi.nlm.nih.gov/pubmed/21900137

Olson-Kennedy J, Rosenthal SM, Hastings J, Wesp L (2016) Health considerations for gender nonconforming children and transgender adolescents. https://transcare.ucsf.edu/guidelines/youth

Pullin Z (2014) Two spirit: the story of a movement unfolds. KOSMOS Journal for Global Transformation. May–June issue. Native Peoples. https://www.kosmosjournal.org/news/two-spirit-the-story-of-a-movement-unfolds/

Rashid M, Sarmad-Tamimy M (2013) Phalloplasty: the dream and the reality. Indian J Plast Surg 46(2):283–293. https://www.ncbi.nlm.nih.gov/pmc/articles/PMC3901910/

Redcay (2015) Transgender issues and eating disorders. June 4, 2018. https://www.edcatalogue.com/transgender-issues-and-eating-disorders/. Accessed 14 Nov 2019

Restar AJ (2018) Methodological Critique of Littman's (2018) Parental-respondents accounts of "rapid-onset" gender dysphoria. Arch Sex Behav 49:61–66. https://doi.org/10.1007/s10508-019-1453-2

Rood BA, Reisner SL, Surace FI, Puckett JA, Maroney MR, Pantalone DW (2016) Expecting rejection: understanding the minority stress experiences of transgender and gender-nonconforming individuals. Transgend Health 1(1):151–164. https://www.ncbi.nlm.nih.gov/pmc/articles/PMC5685272/

Russell ST, Pollitt AM, Li G, Grossman AH (2018) Chosen name use is linked to reduced depressive symptoms, suicidal ideation, and suicidal behavior among transgender youth. J Adolesc Health 63(4):503–505. https://www.jahonline.org/article/S1054-139X(18)30085-5/fulltext#intraref0010a

Sevelius JM (2013) Gender affirmation: a framework for conceptualizing risk behavior among transgender women of color. Sex Roles 68(11–12):675–689. https://www.ncbi.nlm.nih.gov/pmc/articles/PMC3667985/

Spencer MS, Gunter KE, Palmisano G (2010) Community health workers and their value to social work. Soc Work 55(2):169–180. http://chwcentral.org/sites/default/files/Spencer-CHWs%20and%20their%20value%20to%20social%20work.pdf

Stone S (1987) The empire strikes back: a post transsexual manifesto. https://www.semantic-scholar.org/paper/The-Empire-Strikes-Back%3A-A-Posttranssexual-Stone/9b7a007f8cd4166b7faa97b1b4eba208824c28b5

Stryker S (2004/2015) Transgender activism http://www.glbtqarchive.com/ssh/transgender_activism_S.pdf. Accessed 12 Oct 2019

Taylor C (2009) Health and safety issues for aboriginal transgender/two Spirit people in Manitoba. Can J Aboriginal Commun Based HIV/AIDS Res 2:63–84

Taylor JC, Howard-Caldwell C, Baser RE, Faison N, Jackson JS (2007) Prevalence of eating disorders among blacks in the national survey of american life. Int J Eat Disord 40(Suppl):S10–S14. Prevalence of Eating Disorders—Race: https://www.ncbi.nlm.nih.gov/pmc/articles/PMC2882704/

Toomey RB, Anhalt K (2016) Mindfulness as a coping strategy for bias-based school victimization among Latina/o sexual minority youth. Psychol Sex Orientat Gend Divers 3(4):432–441

Trans Student Educational Resources (2019) LGBTQ+ definitions. http://www.transstudent.org/definitions. Accessed 19 Oct 2019

Turban JL, Beckwith N, Reisner SL, Keuroghlian AS (2019) Association between recalled exposure to gender identity conversion efforts and psychological distress and suicide attempts among transgender adults. JAMA Psychiat 77(1):1–9. Online Transgender Women—Conversion Therapy: https://jamanetwork.com/journals/jamapsychiatry/article-abstract/2749479

United States Center for Medicaid & Medicare Services (1989) National coverage determination 140.3: transsexual surgery. 54 Federal Register 34,555, 34,572. https://www.cms.gov/medicare-coverage-database/details/nca-decision-memo.aspx?NCAId=282&CoverageSelection=National&KeyWord=gender+reassignment+surgery&KeyWordLookUp=Title&KeyWordSearchType=And&bc=gAAAACAACAAAAA%3D%3D&

United States Department of Health and Human Services Department (2016) Nondiscrimination in Health Programs and Activities (Section 1557). 81 Federal Register 31375. https://www.federalregister.gov/documents/2016/05/18/2016-11458/nondiscrimination-in-health-programs-and-activities?utm_campaign=subscription+mailing+list&utm_medium=email&utm_source=federalregister.go

University of California, Davis (2019) LGBTQIA resource center glossary. https://lgbtqia.ucdavis.edu/educated/glossary. Accessed 19 Oct 2019

Virupaksha HG, Muralidhar D, Ramakrishna J (2016) Suicide and suicidal behavior among transgender persons. Indian J Psychol Med 38(6):505–509. Suicide and Suicidal Behavior among Transgender Persons: https://www.ncbi.nlm.nih.gov/pmc/articles/PMC5178031/

Wang ED, Kim EA (2016) Postoperative care and common issues after masculinizing chest surgery. https://transcare.ucsf.edu/guidelines/chest-surgery-masculinizing

Williams-Crenshaw K (1994) Mapping the margins: intersectionality, identity politics, and violence against women of color. In: Fineman MA, Mykitiuk R (eds) The public nature of private violence, pp 93–118. https://www.racialequitytools.org/resourcefiles/mapping-margins.pdf

World Professional Association for Transgender Health (2019). https://www.wpath.org. Accessed 23 Sept 2019

Xu H, Kozato A, Fontana S, Pang J, Ting J, Fang F (2019) Complications after breast implant augmentation in a transgender population. J Sci Innov Med 2(2):27. Breast Aug Complications: https://journalofscientificinnovationinmedicine.org/articles/44/

Physical Activity as an Integral Part of Overall Wellness in the College/ Emerging-Adult Population

9

Jacqueline D. Van Hoomissen and Andrew Downs

9.1 PA and Health

It is clear from decades of epidemiological, clinical, and basic science research that physical activity (PA) positively affects health. Engagement in regular PA is associated with a reduced risk for mortality (Paffenbarger et al. 1986; Arem et al. 2015; Lear et al. 2017) and many chronic health conditions (Warburton and Bredin 2017). In addition, PA can also be used as a clinical treatment to improve health for individuals already diagnosed with specific chronic conditions (Pedersen and Saltin 2015). Because of the impressive ability of PA to both prevent negative health outcomes and function as an effective treatment for specific medical conditions, assessment of individual PA levels is now recognized by many health care organizations as an important vital sign, something that should be assessed and monitored throughout the lifespan. Chronic health conditions, sometimes referred to as chronic disease, are illnesses that are not contagious and generally affect an individual over a long period of time. These conditions are now the leading causes of death worldwide and have been on the rise over the last several decades (Anderson and Durstine 2019). The risk for developing many of these conditions is reduced when individuals engage in the recommended levels of PA. The current recommendations from the World Health Organization are 150 min/week of moderate- or 75 min/week of vigorous-intensity PA for adults. PA at these levels reduces the risk for chronic health conditions such as cardiovascular disease, some types of cancer, hypertension, diabetes, dementia, major depression, obesity, stroke, and more. Moving a

J. D. Van Hoomissen (✉)
Department of Biology, University of Portland, Portland, OR, USA
e-mail: vanhoomi@up.edu

A. Downs
Department of Psychological Sciences, University of Portland, Portland, OR, USA
e-mail: downs@up.edu

© Springer Nature Switzerland AG 2021
A. Vermeesch (ed.), *Integrative Health Nursing Interventions for Vulnerable Populations*, https://doi.org/10.1007/978-3-030-60043-3_9

population from less-active to meeting PA guidelines can help prevent unnecessary health burdens at the individual level, which translates to an overall healthier community.

The opposite is also true. When PA levels decline, health declines. It is estimated that more than 25% of adults worldwide are not engaging in sufficient levels of PA (Guthold et al. 2018). The effect is such that if physical inactivity were eliminated, many countries worldwide would see an increase in life expectancy and a decrease in mortality rates for chronic health conditions such as cancer and cardiovascular disease that are the result of physical inactivity (Lee et al. 2012). Efforts to increase individual and community health should focus not only on increasing PA, but simultaneously decreasing physical inactivity or sedentary time.

At a clinical level, PA is an effective treatment for many chronic health conditions and there is evidence that ancient cultures knew this. The writings of the ancient Chinese surgeon, Hua T'O who lived during the East Han Dynasty (25 BCE-250 CE) stated that exercise was important in health and prevented sickness (Tipton 2014). In addition, ancient health practitioners, such as Susruta of India (600 BCE), were aware of the benefits of PA and prescribed it to their patients. This knowledge is now supported with undisputable scientific research that PA and exercise are effective treatments for chronic health conditions, especially when patients are "prescribed" exercise by a practitioner and that prescription outlines the dose of exercise required for maximum benefits. For example, exercise is an effective clinical treatment for reducing symptoms of depression (Blumenthal et al. 2007; Schuch et al. 2016), managing blood glucose in diabetic patients (Colberg et al. 2016), attenuating the progression of coronary artery disease (Winzer et al. 2018), and safely improving the quality of life for patients with breast cancer (Singh et al. 2018). Overall, exercise should be viewed as an integral and necessary part of a holistic treatment plan to improve an individual's health.

9.2   PA Levels in College Students

According to the National Center for Education Statistics (National Center for Education Statistics 2020), individuals transitioning from their teenage years into their emerging adult/early adult years (18–24 years old) currently represent 61% of the United States college student population. This group is at risk for declining PA levels throughout their college years, thus influencing the health habits they carry with them into adulthood. It is important to consider how PA levels have changed over the years within this population but also the historical context in which movement as part of a healthy habit of being was or was not integrated into the US system of higher education.

Beginning in the mid-nineteenth century college professionals began to consider PA an important component of a college education and as integral to the development of the young adults on their campus. In 1861, Amherst College established the first known physical education requirement on a college campus in the United States (Hitchcock 1878). Other colleges quickly followed suit, and by the early 1930s virtually all (i.e., 97%) colleges and universities in the USA had a physical education requirement (McCristal and Miller 1939). Though the exact percentage of colleges requiring physical requirements fluctuated each year thereafter, at least 80% had a physical education requirement through the late 1960s (Lumpkin and Jenkins 1993). Over the next 50 years, mandatory physical education began to disappear from many college campuses such that by 2010 fewer than 40% of colleges and universities required their students to take a physical education course (Cardinal et al. 2012).

Logically, this de-emphasis of PA as an integral part of the college curriculum very well may have led to a decrease in PA in college students over time. However, the lack of epidemiological studies conducted in the nineteenth and much of the twentieth century do not allow for definitive conclusions to be drawn. Indeed, it is theoretically possible that college students may display similar, or perhaps even higher, PA levels in the absence of a specific curricular requirement. Fortunately, in the late twentieth century, researchers began examining PA levels in college students allowing for an examination of PA trends in college students over the past few decades (Douglas et al. 1997).

The Youth Risk Behavior Survey (Kann et al. 1996) is a national US survey that was first administered to high school students in 1995. At that time, 63.7% of high school students reported engaging in vigorous PA for at least 20 min, 3 or more days per week, and 21.1% reported engaging in moderate PA for at least 30 min, 5 or more days per week. The same year, the National College Health Risk Behavior Survey (Douglas et al. 1997) found that only 38% of college students reported engaging in vigorous PA for at least 20 min, 3 or more days per week, and 19.5% reported engaging in moderate PA for at least 30 min, 5 or more days per week. In other words, high school and college students engaged in similar levels of moderate PA, but 25.7% fewer college students engaged in regular vigorous PA when compared to their high school counterparts.

Even more concerning is data suggesting that PA among college students has continued to largely trend downward since that 1995 survey. Specifically, in 2000 the National College Health Assessment (American College Health Association 2000) found that a comparable 40.4% of college students reported engaging in vigorous PA for at least 20 min, 3 or more days per week. However, in the most recent National College Health Assessment survey conducted in 2019 (American College Health Association 2019), only 26.8% of college students reported engaging in vigorous PA for at least 20 min, 3 or more days per week. The lower proportion of college students engaging in vigorous PA at the recommended levels does not appear to have been offset by an increase in moderate PA as only 21.8% of college students in the 2019 NCHA survey reported engaging in moderate PA for at least 30 min, 5 or more days per week. Epidemiological data from national surveys such as the NCHA provide insight into larger population trends which can be verified and examined in more local contexts. Collectively, numerous smaller-scale research studies have also demonstrated decreases in PA in the college student population, with approximately 40–50% of students classified as inactive (Keating et al. 2005).

Such large decreases in vigorous PA from high school to college and over the past 25 years within the college student population suggest that college is very likely a critical transition point for a significant proportion of individuals. Beyond such overall trends, a major question of interest includes how PA patterns change during the college years as students progress from college entry to graduation. Examination of such patterns could produce key insights that may help develop ways of decreasing sedentary time and increasing movement by tailoring interventions to a specific time point in students' college careers. Data from the University Life Study confirmed that college students' daily PA levels decrease as they progress through college, showing a consistent steady decline over seven semesters that results in a significant decrease in activity across the college years for many students (Small et al. 2013).

Taken together, trend data collected in nationwide surveys as well as data from both cross-sectional and longitudinal studies conducted on single campuses provide clear evidence that PA levels are lower in college students than in high school students. In addition, vigorous PA levels among college students have declined significantly over the past 25 years, and a significant proportion of students show a consistent and steady decline in PA as they progress through their college years. These data make clear that college students are a vulnerable population who are at risk for the short-term and long-term health impacts associated with engaging in inadequate PA. These risks are further magnified by the fact that PA typically continues to decline from the age of 24 throughout adulthood (Centers for Disease Control and Prevention 2013).

9.3 Importance of Addressing Declining PA in College Students

Evidence has accumulated over the past few decades that engaging in adequate PA is not only beneficial in improving physical health, it also appears to be a potent protective factor that is linked with a range of improved mental health outcomes. For example, even relatively brief bouts of vigorous PA have been shown to cause decreases in depressive and anxious symptoms (Penedo and Dahn 2005; Adams et al. 2007; Dunn et al. 2001, 2005; Focht et al. 2000; Smith et al. 2007; Wipfli et al. 2008). Indeed, research has consistently demonstrated that PA is an effective treatment for clinical depression and is as effective as FDA-approved medications on the market (Babyak et al. 2000).On a more long-term basis, research suggests that individuals who maintain adequate levels of PA throughout high school and then college experience significantly higher self-esteem, positive emotional states, and lower stress than those who are not active throughout college (Downs and Ashton 2011).

Though it is not completely clear why PA is linked with better mental health (Dishman et al. 2006), there are some possible physiological and psychological mechanisms involved. On the physiological level, researchers have suggested that PA may increase levels of neurotransmitters such as serotonin and norepinephrine, which are believed to play a role in the development of anxious and depressive symptoms for many individuals (Dishman et al. 2000). PA may also reduce levels of stress by decreasing the reactivity of the hypothalamic-pituitary-adrenocortical axis and the amount of cortisol that is released in response to chronic and acute life stressors (Thase et al. 2002). On a psychological level, it appears when individuals are physically active they often experience fewer negative emotions when exposed to stressors and also experience more frequent positive emotions over longer periods of time (Berger and Owen 1998; Dunn and McAuley 2000; Rudolph and Butki 1998).

These findings linking adequate PA with improved mental health are important to consider when thinking about college students because research has demonstrated that a significant proportion of college students report experiencing high levels of stress and are at risk for a range of mental health symptoms. For example, in the 2019 NCHA survey (American College Health Association 2019), student reports indicated that 57.5% felt hopeless, 88% felt overwhelmed, 72% felt very sad, 66.4% felt overwhelming anxiety, 46.2% felt "so depressed that it was difficult to function," and 14.4% seriously considered suicide in the past year. In the same survey, 32.9% of students reported being diagnosed or treated by a professional for a psychological disorder in the past year, 79.6% reported experiencing at least one stressor that was "traumatic or very difficult to handle," and 57.6% reported that they were experiencing higher than average levels of overall stress. Such data clearly indicate that college students are at risk for experiencing high levels of stress and mental health problems. Thus, the positive effects that regular PA can confer on mental health reinforce the importance of working to find ways to increase the PA levels displayed by college students.

In addition to the acute physical and mental health risks associated with inadequate PA during the college years, there is also evidence that the low levels of PA demonstrated by college students may confer risks that extend well into adulthood. The high school and college years have long been conceptualized by psychologists as a critical time for identity development where individuals explore and eventually internalize a sense of who there are as a person (Erikson 1968; Marcia 1994). This sense of identity then helps to direct current and future behavioral choices. For example, if one views themselves as a "dancer," then they will be much more likely to seek out and engage in opportunities to dance than would someone who views themselves as "not a dancer." Research suggests that one component of an individual's identity is whether they view themselves as an "athlete" or an "exerciser," with those who identify as an "athlete" or "exerciser" showing significantly higher levels of PA in high school, college, and adulthood (Downs and Ashton 2011; Anderson et al. 1998).

Not surprisingly, the extent to which individuals view themselves as an "athlete" decreases significantly after the transition to college (Downs and Ashton 2011). This is likely because a much higher proportion of individuals participate in organized sports in high school as compared to college and adulthood. There are exceptions, of course, but if one's perception of themselves as a "non-athlete" or "non-exerciser" becomes part of their identity in college it is believed that they will be less likely to engage in adequate PA in adulthood thus increasing their risk for a host of negative mental and physical health outcomes. There is also evidence that those who engage in adequate PA may do so because they may identify themselves as a "healthy person" as opposed to an "athlete" or "exerciser." Such a "healthy identity" appears to be linked with a range of health-related behaviors including both diet and exercise (Downs and Ashton 2011). In this way, aspects of one's identity related to PA and healthy living that are formed and solidified in college may impact a range of health choices long into the future. Fortunately, it is also believed that if emerging adults are able to increase their PA, they will identify more strongly as an "active" or "healthy" person, again making the college years a critical time for increasing individuals' PA levels.

9.4   Strategies to Increase PA in College Students

When thinking about strategies to increase PA in the college student population, an important first step is to consider taking a holistic and integrative approach to understanding the myriad of factors that collectively combine to influence behavior. Many theoretical models have been developed over the decades to explain the variance in individual and population PA levels based on the interaction of specific factors. The most common models employed generally focus on social, cognitive, or environmental frameworks. Comparing these models' strengths and weaknesses is beyond the scope of this chapter but reviews of the models are available for further study (Center for Disease Control and Prevention 2020; US Department of Health and Human Services President's Council on Sports, Fitness, and Nutrition 2020). The unifying theme in all of these models is that each model includes possible targets for intervention or change that may positively influence behavior. In other situations, however, a lack of attention to a specific influential factor may inadvertently create a barrier to PA participation and this must be taken into account when designing new initiatives.

9.4.1   Policy

One relatively straightforward way to increase PA in the college student population would be for schools to reinstate the mandatory physical education programs that existed from the 1860s through the 1960s. Indeed, it is somewhat curious that while the research evidence showing the widespread benefits of PA for mental and physical health has accumulated, so many higher education institutions have eliminated PA as a requirement (Cardinal et al. 2012). Although some may argue that compulsory PA is not logistically or financially feasible to implement on today's college campuses, it is important to note that, until recently, the vast majority of colleges required PA, and although most today do not, a substantial proportion still do (Cardinal et al. 2012). Incorporating PA into the curriculum in colleges could help bridge the gap between high school and adulthood PA by providing access to the kinds of organized PA programs that so many are exposed to in high school via physical education classes, as well as participation in team sports. Including PA in the college curriculum might also provide opportunities for individuals to experience different forms of PA (e.g., dance, yoga) that they may not have been exposed to yet, and that may be more amenable to long-term engagement in PA than some other forms (e.g., team sports such as football which are not likely to be maintained throughout adulthood).

9.4.2 Built Environment

The built environment is also known to be a factor than can significantly increase or decrease PA levels. A 2016 study (Downs 2016) found that the vast majority of physically active adults cited convenient access to parks and trails and PA facilities as factors that increased their PA moderately to significantly. Perhaps more importantly, these same physically active adults reported that lack of safe places to walk and bike, and lack of access to parks, trails, and exercise facilities were environmental factors that decreased their PA levels (Downs 2016). These findings have clear implications for colleges that wish to increase PA levels in their students. Well-lighted and dedicated walking and biking paths that are free from traffic and other hazards should be developed to the fullest extent possible on college campuses and within the surrounding community. While this may be challenging on some urban campuses, there are certainly a large number of colleges with ample space to create attractive and safe walking and biking paths, as some already choose to do.

Colleges might also consider incentivizing students to walk or bike to campus, rather than driving a car, either through increased parking fees or monetary incentives for those who choose to walk or bike. Colleges could also implement escort programs as part of their work study options, so that students who drive rather than walk due to concerns about personal safety would have the option of having peers safely escort them between campus locations. Having a student recreation center conveniently located on campus and available to students at no, or minimal, cost may also increase PA levels. Some colleges have recently combined their recreation center with another central gathering place for students on campus (e.g., dining services or student union building) in order to coax more students to engage in PA. It is not yet clear whether such placement strategies increase PA, but it certainly would make PA facilities more convenient for at least some students.

9.4.3 Social/Cultural Factors

Research has suggested that there are also several social and cultural factors that could be addressed in order to increase PA levels in college students. For example, physically active adults have reported that using PA as a way to socialize, having friends and romantic partners who support their PA, having friends who are active, and having a workout partner all increase their PA levels (Downs 2016). Of course, colleges cannot ensure that students will have such social supports in place; however, they can take steps to increase the likelihood. For example, providing an array of intramural sports options and group exercise classes can provide students a way to socialize with peers and friends while engaging in PA. Simply requiring PA as part of the curriculum would not only provide students with an opportunity to explore different forms of PA they may enjoy, but would also provide them with an opportunity to form relationships with others in their PA classes around a shared activity that they may engage in together in the future.

Individual interventions. When examining intrapersonal factors that facilitate long-term engagement in PA, Downs (2016) found that the following variables were almost universally cited as increasing PA by physically active adults: enjoying engaging in PA, purposefully planning to engage in PA, valuing PA as part of one's life, thinking being physically active is important, and getting physical and mental health benefits from PA. Indeed, those factors were the only ones of a myriad assessed that were identified by physically active adults as increasing their PA "extremely much."

Such findings have implications for college students who are developing PA patterns that may persist into adulthood. Specifically, colleges should seek to help all of their students understand the importance of PA for maintaining their physical and mental health in order to increase the chances that students will see PA as an important and valuable part of their life. This might occur within the context of traditional PA settings, or in other curricular offerings such as courses that include wellness education and/or a PA component. Colleges should also strive to help students identify the forms of PA they enjoy and how they might plan to engage in those activities more frequently. This, of course, requires that colleges have the built environment and programming that would allow students to easily access their preferred activities.

9.5   Resources for Practitioners

9.5.1   Resources for Additional Information about PA

There are numerous governmental and non-governmental resources available at the national, state, and local level that can assist campus practitioners and partners working to increase PA and healthy lifestyles on their campuses. At the national level, the US Center for Disease Control and Prevention (CDC) website's PA homepage (Center for Disease Control and Prevention 2020) is a leading, authoritative resource that provides readers with PA basics and recommendations for specific populations, summaries of current national initiatives, community and worksite strategies, access to national PA data and statistics, and additional resources. In addition, the US Department of Health and Human Services President's Council on Sports, Fitness, & Nutrition is a federal advisory committee to the CDC. The Council's website provides additional information about national programs and initiatives that can be adopted to promote an active lifestyle (US Department of Health and Human Services President's Council on Sports, Fitness, and Nutrition 2020).

State Departments of Health as well as community-level organizations are also key resources for college campuses as these organizations target their programs to the needs of the local populations and they can be one of many allies who can help support campus initiatives as they are developed and sustained.

Non-governmental organizations are additional valuable resources for the campus PA practitioner. These organizations are often referred to as professional societies, alliances, partnerships, and advocacy groups and each has a unique mission that guides their work. The American College of Sports Medicine (American College of Sports Medicine 2020) is a professional organization of over 50,000 members from around the world who are dedicated to using scientific research to support health education and advocacy focused on PA. Through this organization many campus stakeholders can engage in ongoing continuing education, pursue PA certifications, and use ACSM's policy and position statements to bolster support for new initiatives. The National PA Plan Alliance (National Physical Activity Plan Alliance 2020) is an organization of stakeholders across many sectors of society who work together to promote the National PA Plan. This plan contains specific college and university tactics that can be used to guide program development. These tactics range from creation of PA courses required for graduation to making campus PA goals part of the institution's long-term strategic plan.

9.5.2 Resources for Initiating a New Program to Address PA Levels

For those practitioners on campus who are at the initial stages of assessing how their current PA programing and recreational facilities support their overall goals of improving health should consider completing a campus audit as a first step in strategizing where and how to invest resources. The *PA Campus Environmental Supports* (PACES) audit is a validated method for examining 11 aspects of campus operations including programing, the built environment, marketing, staffing, access, and more (Horacek et al. 2019). The data gathered from an audit can then be used by all stakeholders across campus as baseline information that can continually be re-examined as campuses further develop their programs and facilities. Data from an audit can also be combined with campus health surveys that focus on individual behavior and attitudes. One such survey is the National College Health Association's National College Health Assessment survey (National College Health Association's National College Health Assessment 2020) which provides detailed information about students' health habits, behaviors, and perceptions.

Campus leaders may develop as part of their new programs, a method that can be used to measure their students' PA levels. There are many validated measures/methods used today in both research and public/community health settings. These measures are generally categorized as self-report measures involving questionnaires, objective measures that utilize technology, such as accelerometers/pedometers/bands and other monitors, and criterion-based measures that are more physiologically based and require lab equipment to perform. No method perfectly measures

PA given the inability for any one measure or method to capture all aspects of a complex behavior and the challenge to fully and accurately assess it in free-living situations, which is typical in the college student population. Nevertheless, measures do exist that can help capture meaningful data for program development, implementation, and continued surveillance of program goals (Dowd et al. 2018; Sylvia et al. 2014).

When choosing a method of PA assessment, practitioners should first consider determining which data points are most important to capture and how these data will enhance their work, making it more meaningful and sustainable. Beginning with an examination of numerous methods available will help practitioners determine which method aligns best with their goals. Questions to consider before initiating the review of methods are: (1) Am I interested in a general measure of whether students meet nationally recommended guidelines? (e.g., CDC guidelines for PA), (2) Am I interested in capturing more specific aspects of PA? (e.g., how frequently participants engage in PA, duration of each bout of PA, types of exercise performed), (3) How often do I plan on measuring PA and what method is both valid and reliable but also *feasible* within my population? (e.g., quick surveys distributed through social media vs. technology-based methods that require in person contact with each participant). The importance of feasibility of a measure is a critical consideration as the value of the chosen method is only as good as its ability to implement for the duration of a program. Overall, self-report surveys/questionnaires/diaries are very feasible to implement but may not capture accurately the duration of activities and/or the intensity, which may be better assessed using object methods that utilize technology such as accelerometers. These objective measures, however, may not be able to capture the qualitative nature of PA (e.g., playing sports, running, walking to the store) that is best captured through self-report. Regardless of the limitations of all methods, practitioners interested in creating programs to increase PA levels in their communities are strongly encouraged to identify at least one assessment method that can be used during the duration of the school's endeavors in this area.

Once programs are well established and supported, institutions may want to consider receiving national recognition for their efforts as a way to further establish and sustain their work. In 2014, ACSM launched its Exercise is Medicine on Campus recognition program (Exercise is Medicine on Campus 2020) that calls on college campuses to support campus health and well-being through a commitment to making movement a part of everyone's daily routine, instituting PA assessment as part of every campus health center, creating a referral system for at-risk students in need of expert fitness support to change behavior, providing resources for students to improve their PA levels.

9.6   Summary and Conclusions

Campus environments are key players in promoting PA and overall community health. Creating conditions that promote adoption of healthy behaviors while simultaneously reducing barriers requires collaboration across many areas of campus operation from academic to student services to community partners. An integrative approach allows for multiple factors to be incorporated in creating a campus environment aimed at optimizing wellness for emerging adults.

References

Adams TB, Moore MT, Dye J (2007) The relationship between physical activity and mental health in a national sample of college females. Women Health 45(1):69–85. https://doi.org/10.1300/J013v45n01_05

American College Health Association (2000) American College Health Association-National College Health Assessment: Reference Group Executive Summary Spring 2000. American College Health Association, Baltimore. https://www.acha.org/NCHA/ACHA-NCHA_Data/Publications_and_Reports/NCHA/Data/Publications_and_Reportsaspx?hkey=d5fb767c-d15d-4efc-8c41-3546d92032c5. Accessed 19 May 2020

American College Health Association (2019) American College Health Association-National College Health Assessment II: Undergraduate Student Executive Summary Spring 2019. American College Health Association, Silver Spring, MD. https://www.acha.org/NCHA/ACHA-NCHA_Data/Publications_and_Reports/NCHA/Data/Publications_and_Reportsaspx?hkey=d5fb767c-d15d-4efc-8c41-3546d92032c5. Accessed 19 May 2020

American College of Sports Medicine (2020). http://www.acsm.org. Accessed 13 Apr 2020

Anderson E, Durstine JL (2019) PA, exercise, and chronic diseases: a brief review. Sports Med Health Sci 1:3–10. https://doi.org/10.1016/j.smhs.2019.08.006

Anderson DF, Cychosz CM, Franke WD (1998) Association of exercise identity with measures of exercise commitment and physiological indicators of fitness in a law enforcement cohort. J Sport Behav 21(3):233–241

Arem H, Moore SC, Patel A, Hartge P, Berrington de Gonzalez A, Visvanathan K et al (2015) Leisure time PA and mortality: a detailed pooled analysis of the dose-response relationship. JAMA Intern Med 175(6):959–967. https://doi.org/10.1001/jamainternmed.2015.0533

Babyak M, Blumenthal JA, Herman S et al (2000) Exercise treatment for major depression: maintenance of therapeutic benefit at 10 months. Psychosom Med 62(5):633–638

Berger BG, Owen DR (1998) Relation of low and moderate intensity exercise with acute mood change in college joggers. Percept Mot Skills 87(2):611–621

Blumenthal JA, Babyak MA, Doraiswamy PM et al (2007) Exercise and pharmacotherapy in the treatment of major depressive disorder. Psychosom Med 69:587–596. https://doi.org/10.1097/PSY.0b013e318148c19a

Cardinal BJ, Sorensen SD, Cardinal MK (2012) Historical perspective and current status of the physical education graduation requirement at American 4-year colleges and universities. Res Q Exerc Sport 83(4):503–512. https://doi.org/10.1080/02701367.2012.10599139

Center for Disease Control and Prevention (2020). https://www.cdc.gov/physicalactivity/. Accessed 13 Apr 2020

Centers for Disease Control and Prevention (2013) Adult participation in aerobic and muscle-strengthening physical activities—United States, 2011. MMWR 62:326–300

Colberg SR, Sigal RJ, Yardley JE, Riddell MC, Dunstan DW, Dempsey PC et al (2016) Physical activity/exercise and diabetes: a position statement of the American Diabetes Association. Diabetes Care 39:2065–2079. https://doi.org/10.2337/dc16-1728

Dishman RK, Renner KJ, White-Welkley JE, Burke KA, Bunnell BN (2000) Treadmill exercise training augments brain norepinephrine response to familiar and novel stress. Brain Res Bull 52(5):337–342

Dishman RK, Berthoud H-R, Booth FW et al (2006) Neurobiology of exercise. Obesity (Silver Spring) 14(3):345–356. https://doi.org/10.1038/oby.2006.46

Douglas KA, Collins JL, Warren CW, Kann L, Gold R, Clayton S (1997) Results from the 1995 National College Health Risk Behavior Survey. J Am Coll Health 46:55–66. https://doi.org/10.1080/07448489709595589

Dowd K, Szeklicki R, Minetto MA, Murphy MH, Polito A, Ghigo E et al (2018) A systematic literature review of reviews on techniques for physical activity measurement in adults: a DEDIPAC study. Int J Behav Nutr Phys Act 15(1):15. https://doi.org/10.1186/s12966-017-0636-2

Downs A (2016) Physically active adults: an analysis of the key variables that keep them moving. Am J Health Educ 47(5):299–308

Downs A, Ashton J (2011) Vigorous physical activity, sports participation, and athletic identity: implications for mental and physical health in college students. J Sport Behav 34(3):228–249

Dunn EC, McAuley E (2000) Affective responses to exercise bouts of varying intensities. J Soc Behav Pers 15(2):201–214

Dunn AL, Trivedi MH, O'Neal HA (2001) PA dose-response effects on outcomes of depression and anxiety. Med Sci Sports Exerc 33(6 Suppl):S587–S597

Dunn AL, Trivedi MH, Kampert JB, Clark CG, Chambliss HO (2005) Exercise treatment for depression: efficacy and dose response. Am J Prev Med 28(1):1–8. https://doi.org/10.1016/j.amepre.2004.09.003

Erikson E (1968) Identity: youth and crisis. Norton, New York

Exercise is Medicine on Campus (2020). https://www.exerciseismedicine.org/support_page.php/-on-campus/. Accessed 13 Apr 2020

Focht BC, Koltyn KF, Bouchard LJ (2000) State anxiety and blood pressure responses following different resistance exercise sessions. Int J Sport Psychol 31(3):376–390

Guthold R, Stevens GA, Riley LM, Bull FC (2018) Worldwide trends in insufficient PA from 2001 to 2016: a pooled analysis of 358 population-based surveys with 1·9 million participants. Lancet Glob Health 6:e1077–e1e86. https://doi.org/10.1155/2012/546459

Hitchcock E (1878) Hygiene at Amherst College: experience of the Department of Physical Education and Hygiene in Amherst College for the past sixteen years. Public Health Pap Rep 4:46–56

Horacek T, Yildirim ED, Seidman D, Byrd-Bredbenner C, Colby S (2019) Redesign, field-testing, and validation of the physical activity campus environmental supports (PACES) audit. J Environ Public Health. https://doi.org/10.1155/2019/5819752

Kann L., Warren CW, Harris MM, Collins JL, Williams BI (1996) Youth risk behavior surveillance—United States, 1995. https://www.cdc.gov/mmwr/preview/mmwrhtml/00043812.htm. Accessed 8 Jan 2020

Keating X, Guan J, Pinero J, Bridges D (2005) A meta-analysis of college students' physical activity behaviors. J Am Coll Health 54(2):166–125. https://doi.org/10.3200/JACH.54.2.116-126

Lear SA, Hu W, Rangarajan S, Gasevic D, Leong D, Iqbal R et al (2017) The effect of PA on mortality and cardiovascular disease in 130 000 people from 17 high-income, middle-income, and low-income countries: the PURE study. Lancet 390:2643–2654. https://doi.org/10.1177/1090198112467801

Lee I-M, Shiroma EJ, Lobelo F, Puska P, Blair SN, Katzmarzyk PT (2012) Effect of physical inactivity on major non-communicable diseases worldwide: an analysis of burden of disease and life expectancy. Lancet 380:219–229. https://doi.org/10.1016/S0140-6736(12)61031-9

Lumpkin A, Jenkins J (1993) Basic instruction programs: a brief history. J Phys Educ Recreat Dance 64(6):33–36. https://doi.org/10.1080/07303084.1993.10609999

Marcia JE (1994) The empirical study of ego identity. In: Bosma HA, Graafsma TLG, Grotevant HD, de Levita DJ (eds) Identity and development: an interdisciplinary approach. Sage, Thousand Oaks, CA

McCristal KJ, Miller EA (1939) A brief survey of the preset status of the health and physical education requirements for men students in colleges and universities. Res Q 10(4):70–80ii

National Center for Education Statistics (2020). http://nces.ed.gov. Accessed 13 Apr 2020

National College Health Association's National College Health Assessment (2020). https://www.acha.org/NCHA/NCHA_Home. Accessed 13 Apr 2020

National Physical Activity Plan Alliance (2020). http://www.physicalactivityplan.org/index.html. Accessed 13 Apr 2020

Paffenbarger RS, Hyde RT, Wing AL, Hsieh CC (1986) Physical activity, all-cause mortality, and longevity of college alumni. N Engl J Med 314:6015–6013

Pedersen BK, Saltin B (2015) Exercise as medicine—evidence for prescribing exercise as therapy in 26 different chronic diseases. Scand J Med Sci Sports 25:1–72. https://doi.org/10.1111/sms.12581

Penedo FJ, Dahn JR (2005) Exercise and well-being: a review of mental and physical health benefits associated with PA. Curr Opin Psychiatry 18(2):189–193

Rudolph DL, Butki BD (1998) Self-efficacy and affective responses to short bouts of exercise. J Appl Sport Psychol 10(2):268–280. https://doi.org/10.1080/10413209808406393

Schuch FB, Vancampfort D, Richards J, Rosenbaum S, Ward PB, Stubbs B (2016) Exercise as a treatment for depression: a meta-analysis adjusting for publication bias. J Psychiatr Res 77:42–51. https://doi.org/10.1016/j.jpsychires.2016.02.023

Singh B, Spence RR, Steele ML, Sandler CX, Peake JM, Hayes SC (2018) A systematic review and meta-analysis of the safety, feasibility, and effect of exercise in women with stage II+ breast cancer. Arch Phys Med Rehabil 99:2621–2636. https://doi.org/10.1016/j.apmr.2018.03.026

Small M, Bailey-Davis L, Morgan N, Maggs J (2013) Changes in eating and PA behaviors across seven semesters of college: living on or off campus matters. Health Educ Behav 40(4):435–441. https://doi.org/10.1177/1090198112467801

Smith PJ, Blumenthal JA, Babyak MA, Georgiades A, Hinderliter A, Sherwood A (2007) Effects of exercise and weight loss on depressive symptoms among men and women with hypertension. J Psychosom Res 63(5):463–469. https://doi.org/10.1016/j.jpsychores.2007.05.011

Sylvia LG, Bernstein EE, Hubbard JL, Keating L, Anderson EJ (2014) Practical guide to measuring physical activity. J Acad Nutr Diet 114(2):199–208. https://doi.org/10.1016/j.jand.2013.09.018

Thase ME, Jindal R, Howland RH (2002) Biological aspects of depression. In: Gotlib IH, Hammen CL (eds) Handbook of depression. The Guilford Press, New York, NY, pp 192–218

Tipton CM (2014) The history of "exercise is medicine" in ancient civilizations. Adv Physiol Educ 38(2):109–117. https://doi.org/10.1152/advan.00136.2013

US Department of Health and Human Services President's Council on Sports, Fitness, & Nutrition (2020). https://www.hhs.gov/fitness/be-active/index.html. Accessed 13 Apr 2020

Warburton DER, Bredin SSD (2017) Health benefits of PA: a systematic review of current systematic reviews. Curr Opin Cardiol 32:541–556. https://doi.org/10.1097/HCO.0000000000000437

Winzer EB, Woitek F, Linke A (2018) Physical activity in the prevention and treatment of coronary artery disease. J Am Heart Assoc 7. https://doi.org/10.1161/JAHA.117.007725

Wipfli BM, Rethorst CD, Landers DM (2008) The anxiolytic effects of exercise: a meta-analysis of randomized trials and dose-response analysis. J Sport Exerc Psychol 30(4):392–410

Physical Activity Interventions Among African American Women

10

Wanda M. Williams

10.1 Introduction

Engaging in regular physical activity (PA), defined as at least 150 min of moderate intensity weekly, can improve overall health and fitness, and lower the risk for many chronic diseases, such as heart disease, some cancers, stroke, obesity, and Type 2 diabetes (US Department of Health and Human Services 2018). Yet, the percentage of African American women meeting federal physical activity guidelines of engaging in moderate physical activity for ≥150 min/week was 39% compared to 54% in White women and 42% in Hispanic women (Benjamin Emelia et al. 2019). African American women consistently report lowest level of physical activity than other ethnic/racial groups (Lee, 2010).

The top four causes of death for African American women are coronary heart disease, cancer, stroke, and diabetes, in that order (US Department of Health and Human Services, 2010). Contributing factors for these diseases are multifaceted; however, low engagement in physical activity and sedentary behavior have been linked to the growing incidence of these diseases in African American women. Low physical activity begins to be evident in preadolescent African American females and continues across the lifespan (Webb et al. 2016).

Statistical data reveals that African American women have higher prevalence of high blood pressure, cardiovascular disease (CVD), stroke, and heart failure than any other ethnic group (Benjamin Emelia et al. 2019). Table 10.1 shows the prevalence noted among females from different ethnic/racial backgrounds as it related to various health conditions. As evident by the statistical data in the table, African American women have higher prevalence of all of these health conditions expected for diagnosed diabetes. Evidence support that the morbidity and mortality

W. M. Williams (✉)
Rutgers School of Nursing—Camden, Camden, NJ, USA
e-mail: wanda.williams@rutgers.edu

© Springer Nature Switzerland AG 2021
A. Vermeesch (ed.), *Integrative Health Nursing Interventions for Vulnerable Populations*, https://doi.org/10.1007/978-3-030-60043-3_10

Table 10.1 Comparison of selected health conditions among females of different ethnic/racial backgrounds (%) (Benjamin Emelia et al. 2019)

Health conditions	Asian	White	Hispanic	African American
Overweight (BMI $\geq$ 25.0 kg/m^2)	34.6	63.7	77.1	82.2
Obese (BMI $\geq$ 30.0 kg/m^2)	11.9	35.5	45.7	56.9
High blood pressure (HBP)	36.4	41.3	40.8	56.0
Cardiovascular disease (CVD)	37.2	43.4	42.6	57.1
Heart failure	0.7	1.9	2.1	3.9
Diagnosed diabetes	9.9	7.3	14.1	13.4
Stroke	1.6	2.5	2.2	3.8

BMI (body mass index)

associated with these health conditions can be significantly reduced with regular physical activity (Knight, 2012; World Health Organization, 2014; Centers for Disease Control and Prevention, 1999).

10.2 Healthy People

Healthy People is a program aimed at health promotion and disease prevention, with 10-year targets to guide and improve the health of all people in the United States based on evidence-based goals and objectives (HP 2010, 2000). Physical activity has ranked as a leading health indicator since Healthy People launch in 1979 and as we approach Healthy People 2030, physical activity is still recognized as an essential factor in disease prevention and health promotion (Healthy People 2030, 2019). Healthy People reflects a multidisciplinary approach to promoting physical activity through policies and programs that looks at transportation, urban planning, recreation, environmental health, and other fields. Healthy people 2020 met its target to "*increase the proportion of adults who engage in aerobic physical activity of at least moderate intensity for at least 150 minutes/week, or 75 minutes/ week of vigorous intensity, or an equivalent combination*" (HP 2020, 2017). Although healthy people 2020 population goals have been met, level of physical activity of African American women still remains lower than all other groups (Benjamin Emelia et al. 2019). The benefits to regular physical activity have been established; and regular physical activity could significantly reduce the health disparities noted among African American women. Therefore, interventions targeted for African American women are required to get and keep this segment of the population moving.

10.3 Integrative Healthcare (IHC)

Incorporating physical activity programs or educational information about physical activity into a person's life would be an essential component in Integrative healthcare (IHC). Integrative healthcare is an important approach to care that considers multiple aspects to providing and developing healthcare to patients (Leach et al. 2018). Nurses as part of the healthcare team play an important role in providing information on implementation and benefits of maintaining a lifestyle that include being physically active.

10.4   Cultural Considerations

Statistics show that physical inactivity is higher in African American women than in other ethnic/racial groups (Benjamin Emelia et al. 2019; Lee et al. 2012), but a clear explanation for these differences is unknown. A key significant factor for the lack of physical activity among African American women may rest with cultural beliefs and attitudes. Culture has been identified as a key factor on health behavior and decision making (Boyington et al. 2008; Resnicow et al. 1999; Joseph et al. 2016) and is defined as a set of beliefs, values, attitudes, role perceptions, and customs that are shared among a group of people (Corneille et al. 2005). Therefore, culture influences need to be considered when attempting to change health behavior and attitudes related to physical activity among African American women. Physical activity programs that are more culturally tailored may be more effective (Joseph et al. 2016; Baskin et al. 2015).

A cultural factor that influences participation in physical activity among African American women is hair maintenance. Hair maintenance is an important issue with African American women when it comes to being physically active. Current research indicates that Black hair care maintenance may be a significant deterrent to being physically active (Martin 2012; Williams et al. 2017; Huebschmann et al. 2016). Gabby Douglas (2012 London Olympic) and Simone Biles (2016 Rio Olympic) both gold-medal winners in gymnastics received unwanted attention and criticism of their hair during their Olympic performances (Hudson 2016). The texture of Black women hair varies, and heat and sweat can cause various maintenance concerns, leading to very lengthy hours and extensive cost to fix, with most African American women complaining that physical activity is not worth the amount of time and money to redo their hair (Williams et al. 2017). In 2011, the Surgeon General of the United States, Dr. Regina Benjamin, advocated for Black women to put their health and well-being before their hair—Stating, *"Don't Let Hair Get In The Way of your Health"* (Martin, 2012). Dr. Benjamin emphasized that not only could excess weight, obesity, diabetes, hypertension, and stokes be significantly reduced with regular physical activity, but so could the economic burden that these diseases places on society (Martin, 2012).

Physical inactivity in African American women can also be associated with attitude. A person's attitude is shaped by their experiences, beliefs, and cultural influences (Boyington et al. 2008; Ajzen et al. 2007). Attitude is defined as the individual's positive or negative feelings about performing a behavior, such as being physically active. Some studies have shown that attitudes toward physical activity is an important predictor of engaging in physical activity (James et al. 2014; Poobalan et al. 2012; Nelson et al. 2010).

African American women tend to have a more tolerant attitude toward being a little overweight, referring to themselves as thick, healthy, and big boned, believing big-is-beautiful (Boyington et al. 2008; Deforche et al. 2006; Thompson 2011). Although this attitude indicates a more positive self-image, it negates the need to engage in regular physical activity (Boyington et al. 2008; Thompson, 2011; Barr-Anderson et al. 2008). Qualitative studies by Boyington et al. (2008) and Mabry et al. (2003) supported this concept that African American women were more accepting and satisfied with their body image of fuller hips and rounded buttocks.

Based on these cultural considerations, physical activity interventions directed at African American women would need to incorporate these factors when designing and implementing physical activity interventions among this group.

10.5 Physical Activity Interventions Among African American Women

This section will provide a brief overview of intervention strategies that have shown to be the most effective when promoting physical activity among African American women. The physical activity intervention strategies will be discussed based on identified barriers to physical activity for African American women. Barriers or factors identified by African American women that prevents or hinders their engagement in regular physical activity are hair maintenance, costs, childcare/caregiving, unsafe surroundings, and lack of time (Webb et al. 2016; Jenkins et al. 2017; Bland and Sharma, 2017).

A systematic review of physical activity interventions for African American women was conducted by Bland and Sharma (2017). In their review they identified 13 interventions with most, if not all outcomes aimed at increasing physical activity. Strategies in these interventions included problem-solving, faith-based, social support, goal setting, and group activities (Bland and Sharma, 2017). A similar review of African American women regarding promoting physical activity was conducted by Jenkins et al. (2017) which included 32 studies; however, physical activity was not the main outcome for many of the studies. The intervention strategies included in Jenkins et al. review included culturally tailored interventions, faith-based interventions, group-based programs, and individually tailored programs (Jenkins et al. 2017); other strategies included face-to-face sessions, telephone sessions, a combination of face-to-face and telephone sessions, and peer support (Jenkins et al. 2017).

The phrase *culturally tailored interventions* appears in many of these studies. Care should be taken to ensure that interventions are truly culturally tailored. Culturally tailored strategies should incorporate *surface and deep structure* material, information, and messaging. Examples of surface structure include matching intervention materials and messages to observable characteristics of the population of interest, such as commonly used products (music, food, and clothing), behavior patterns, and environmental and social contexts in which behaviors occur (Barrera Jr. et al. 2013). Deep structure refers to programs that reflect ways by which culture, social, psychological, environmental, and historical factors and values can influence behavior, and particularly how these factors influence behaviors across different population subgroups (Barrera Jr. et al. 2013).

10.6 Specific Interventions

For the purpose of this chapter, only randomized controlled trials (RCT) conducted among African American women were considered to ensure a true cause-effect relationship between the intervention and outcomes. Five RCT of physical activity interventions among African American Women will be reviewed that highlight the importance of social support among this group as well as other key components, such as faith-based, tailored programs and motivational interviewing:

1. The *home-based individually tailored physical activity print (HIPP)* intervention was a randomized controlled trial conducted by Pekmezi et al. (2018), aimed at African American women ($N = 84$) in the Deep South. HIPP was a 12-month physical activity and psychosocial intervention that encouraged participants to gradually increase their physical activity level until national recommendations were met (Pekmezi et al. 2018). The intervention involved motivational matched physical activity manuals with individually tailored feedback reports. The intervention was underpinned by the social cognitive theory and the transtheoretical model. Other components of the intervention included: Self-efficacy (confidence in one's ability to be active despite barriers), decisional balance (weighing the pros and cons of participating in physical activity), social support from friends and family for physical activity, anticipated consequences of physical activity, perceived enjoyment of physical activity, and self-regulation [physical activity goal setting and planning] (Pekmezi et al. 2018). Participants in the HIPP intervention arm increased their self-reported MVPA from 35.1 min/week (SD = 47.8) at baseline to 124 min/week (SD = 95.5) at 12 months, compared with the control participants who reported increases from 48.2 min/week (SD = 51.3) to 102.5 min/week (SD = 94.5) over 12 months (between-group $p > 0.05$). The largest gains in MVPA occurred during the active intervention phase, with the HIPP arm reporting an approximate 33 min/week greater increase in physical activity from baseline to 6 months than the wellness contact control arm (between-group $p > 0.05$). The study protocol also studied the long-term impact of physical activity interventions 12 months after the tapered intervention phase [months 6–12] (Pekmezi et al. 2018). The HIPP intervention addressed the barriers of cost, time, and childcare, since the intervention was conducted in the home and required minimal effort on the part of the participants. The HIPP intervention also included social support which is an important factor among African American women (Jenkins et al. 2017; Reed et al. 2017).
2. *The Sisters in Motion* was a faith-based intervention conducted over 8 weeks for 90 min (Duru et al. 2010). Participants ($N = 62$) were African American women

aged 60 and older who were sedentary. The 8-week intervention curriculum incorporated evidence-based best practice approaches for physical activity programs targeting older adults, including providing activity choices and positive reinforcement, enhancing self-efficacy, and building social support for exercise (Duru et al. 2010). Classes were led by fitness instructor or research assistant. Activities included walking, resistance and balance exercises, as well as line dancing, praise dancing to spiritual music, and basic yoga. At 6 months, intervention participants had increased their weekly steps by 9883 on average, compared with an increase of 2426 for controls ($p = 0.02$); systolic blood pressure (SBP) decreased on average by 12.5 mmHg in intervention participants and only 1.5 mmHg in controls [$p = 0.007$] (Duru et al. 2010). This faith-based approach shows promise in increasing physical activity in this population reinforcing social support and group activities. For many in the Black community, the church and their faith is an important part of their lives (The Barna Group, 2008; Geller et al. 2019), therefore, this faith-based approach has the potential to influence the health of African American women.

3. *The Heart Healthy and Ethnically Relevant Lifestyle trial* was a community-based, culturally relevant intervention to promote healthy eating and physical activity among African American women ($N = 266$) between the ages of 45–65 years (Parra-Medina et al. 2011). Participants were randomized into comprehensive or standard care. The comprehensive group received standard care plus the following: 12 motivational, stage matched, ethnically tailored newsletters over 1 year; an in-depth, introductory telephone call; and up to 14 brief, motivationally tailored telephone counseling calls from research staff over 1 year (Parra-Medina et al. 2011). The telephone counseling addressed a variety of issues, such as safe walking areas, beliefs about food and body image. All material was culturally developed at the surface and deep levels (cultural values, photo, etc.). Data collection was matched to already existing clinic visit to reduce travel burden on participants. Primary outcomes were 6- and 12-month self-reported physical activity and dietary fat intake. The comprehensive intervention improved women's leisure time physical activity (OR = 3.82; 95% CI = 1.41, 10.3) at 6 months (no 12-month differences) (Parra-Medina et al. 2011). This model could be replicated by other primary care providers emphasizing the importance of lifestyle counseling. This intervention addressed the barriers of cost, time, and support by scheduling interviews and data collection with already scheduled appointments; providing telephone counseling that addressed concerns and problem solved for issues hindered a participant from being physically active.

4. The *Women's Lifestyle Physical Activity program* was an RCT of African American women that included a 24-week active intervention period followed by a 24-week maintenance intervention period [total 48 weeks] (Wilbur et al. 2015). The behavior theory for this study was the social cognitive theory. The program had a core component and tested 3 intervention conditions: (1) a person-administered telephone contact; (2) an automated telephone contact; and (3) no telephone contact as the control condition (Wilbur et al. 2015). The core, deliv-

ered in all conditions, included a physical activity prescription and six group meetings held at the community healthcare site. The physical activity prescription was tailored to the individual woman with a goal to increase the eventual number of steps walked to 3000 steps over her baseline steps. Each woman received an accelerometer and entered her steps weekly into an automated telephone computer linked system (Wilbur et al. 2015). Group time was spent emphasizing self-management. Discussion in group meetings held during the active intervention focused on increasing lifestyle physical activity, dealing with personal and environmental problems that can interfere with physical activity, and handling relapses to a more sedentary lifestyle. The two telephone (motivational interviewing) contact approaches were tailored to the individual and intended to sustain effects between group meetings. Adherence to physical activity increased significantly. Group meetings were a powerful intervention for increasing physical activity and preventing weight gain. This model supports the importance of social support in the form of the group meetings as well as the motivational telephone calls.

5. An *8-week individualized, home-based program* to examine the effect of lifestyle physical activity (LPA) on blood pressure in sedentary African American women aged 18–45 years was conducted by Staffileno et al. (2007). Women was randomized to an *Exercise* ($n = 14$) group with instruction to engage in lifestyle-compatible physical activity (e.g., walking, stair climbing) for 10 min, three times a day, 5 days a week, at a prescribed heart rate corresponding to an intensity of 50–60% heart rate reserve (Staffileno et al. 2007). Women in the *No Exercise* group ($n = 10$) were instructed to continue their usual daily activities. Lifestyle physical activity is the accumulation of at least 30 min of self-selected activities (including leisure, occupational, or household activities) performed at a level of moderate intensity, which may be planned or unplanned, and incorporated as part of everyday life. The goal of the intervention was to accumulate 150 min of physical activity per week, which is the minimum physical activity guidelines recommended by the federal government. A private 60-min education session held for the intervention group and the following topics were reviewed: (1) health benefits of LPA, (2) safety issues, (3) goal setting and self-monitoring, (4) identifying physical activity barriers and developing strategies to overcome them, (5) identifying simple ways to incorporate activity into daily living, and (6) creating ways to individualize physical activity (Staffileno et al. 2007). Women were instructed to keep a log documenting physical activity mode, frequency, duration, and heart rate. In addition, participants were shown how to use and wear a portable heart rate monitor. The main focus during the education session was to identify ways to easily incorporate physical activity into daily living. Women randomized to the *No Exercise* group were instructed to continue with their usual daily activities. Activity logs and heart rate monitors were not used with the No Exercise group. The Exercise group had a significant reduction in systolic blood Pressure (SBP) (-6.4 mmHg, $p = 0.036$) and a reduction in diastolic blood pressure (DBP) [-3.3 mmHg] (Staffileno et al. 2007). This study reinforces the importance of tailoring behavior change interventions to meet

culture-specific, sex-specific, and age-specific needs of a target population, such as middle-aged African American women. The results of this study also highlight the significance of regular physical activity as an important intervention for reducing cardiovascular risk more highly prevalent in African American women.

When considering nursing interventions regarding these studies and the role they can play in promoting physical activity. Nurses can educate women about how to safely start or implement physical activity into their daily lives, and how to continue and maintain being physically active; helping patients to set goals, identifying, and addressing barriers to physical activity. Nurses should be aware of the benefits associated with physical activity that leads to the reduction of morbidity associated with chronic diseases. Nurses can follow up with motivational telephone calls or offer encouragement to patients during the intake period at office visits. Practical information on various forms of physical activity should be readily available to patient at most, if not all clinical settings.

10.7   Implications for Future Studies

Physical activity interventions should target health habits and personal behaviors that affect an individual's ability to be physically active. Future research aimed at African American women must develop sustainable, practical, and culturally tailored physical activity programs. Based on the interventions presented in this chapter, behavioral components (use behavioral theories) to understand the perceptions of the lack of physical activity among African American women need to be incorporated in physical activity intervention for this population.

Social support is an important factor for most African American woman, therefore more programs need to be available in their communities that support and encourage a more active lifestyle. More public policies need to be initiated around physical activity especially in regard to the built environment to ensure safe walkable communities.

10.8   Conclusion

Regular physical activity enhances the quality of life for people of all ages. Evidence show that active people outlive those who are inactive. A key role of nurses in promoting physical activity would be that of educator and to support patients' efforts to start and maintain physical activity programs. Physical activity would be an essential factor in integrative healthcare (IHC), considering that being physically active is an important aspect of overall health and recognized as essential for the primary prevention of chronic diseases. Physical activity is considered an economic and low-cost alternative to treating chronic diseases. For African American women being more physically active may be the key to improved health and an effective way to reduce the health disparity observed among African American women.

References

Ajzen I, Albarracin D, Hornik R (eds) (2007) Prediction and change of health behavior. Lawrence Erlbaum Associates, Mahwah, NJ

Barr-Anderson DJ, Neumark-Stzainer DR, Schmitz KH, Ward DS, Conway T, Pratt C et al (2008) But I like PE: factors associated with enjoyment of physical education class in middle school girls. Res Q Exerc Sport 79(1):18–27

Barrera M Jr, Castro FG, Strycker LA, Toobert DJ (2013) Cultural adaptations of behavioral health interventions: a progress report. J Consult Clin Psychol 81(2):196–205. https://doi.org/10.1037/a0027085

Baskin ML, Dulin-Keita A, Thind H, Godsey E (2015) Social and cultural environment factors influencing physical activity among African-American adolescents. J Adolesc Health 56(5):536–542. https://doi.org/10.1016/j.jadohealth.2015.01.012

Benjamin Emelia J, Muntner P, Alonso A, Bittencourt Marcio S, Callaway Clifton W, Carson April P et al (2019) Heart disease and stroke statistics—2019 update: a report from the American Heart Association. Circulation 139(10):e56–e528. https://doi.org/10.1161/CIR.0000000000000659

Bland V, Sharma M (2017) Physical activity interventions in African American women: a systematic review. Health Promot Perspect 7(2):52–59. https://doi.org/10.15171/hpp.2017.11

Boyington JE, Carter-Edwards L, Piehl M, Hutson J, Langdon D, McManus S (2008) Culture attitudes toward weight, diet, and physical activity among overweight African American girls. Prev Chronic Dis 5(2):1–9

Centers for Disease Control and Prevention (1999) A report of the surgeon general – physical activity and health: the link between physical activity and morbidity and mortality. Centers for Disease Control and Prevention: US Department of Health and Human Services, Sports TPsCoPFa

Corneille M, Ashcraft A, Belgrave F (2005) What's culture got to do with it? Prevention programs for African American adolescent girls. J Health Care Poor Underserved 16:38

Deforche B, De Bourdeaudhuij I, Tanghe A (2006) Attitude toward physical activity in normal-weight, overweight and obese adolescents. J Adolesc Health 38(5):560–568

Duru OK, Sarkisian CA, Leng M, Mangione CM (2010) Sisters in motion: a randomized controlled trial of a faith-based physical activity intervention. J Am Geriatr Soc 58(10):1863–1869. https://doi.org/10.1111/j.1532-5415.2010.03082.x

Geller K, Harmon B, Burse N, Strayhorn S (2019) Church-based social support's impact on African-Americans' physical activity and diet varies by support type and source. J Relig Health 58(3):977–991. https://doi.org/10.1007/s10943-018-0576-4

Healthy People 2030 (2019) Healthy People 2030 framework. US Department of Health and Human Services, Office of Disease Prevention and Heath Promotion. https://www.healthypeople.gov/2020/About-Healthy-People/Development-Healthy-People-2030/Framework

HP 2010 (2000) What is healthy people? https://www.healthypeople.gov/. Accessed 19 Dec 2009

HP 2020 (2017) Healthy People 2020: midcourse review. U.S. Department of Health and Human Services. 18 June 2018

Hudson J (2016) Black women, hair and Olympic power. The Undefeated

Huebschmann AG, Campbell LJ, Brown CS, Dunn AL (2016) "My hair or my health:" overcoming barriers to physical activity in African American women with a focus on hairstyle-related factors. Women Health 56(4):428–447. https://doi.org/10.1080/03630242.2015.1101743

James D, Efunbumi O, Harville C, Sears C (2014) Barriers and motivators to physical activity among African American women. Health Educator 46(2):28–34

Jenkins F, Jenkins C, Gregoski MJ, Magwood GS (2017) Interventions promoting physical activity in African American women: an integrative review. J Cardiovasc Nurs 32(1):22–29

Joseph RP, Keller C, Affuso O, Ainsworth BE (2016) Designing culturally relevant physical activity programs for African-American women: a framework for intervention development. J Racial Ethn Health Disparities:1–13. https://doi.org/10.1007/s40615-016-0240-1

Knight JA (2012) Physical inactivity: associated diseases and disorders. Ann Clin Lab Sci 42(3):320–337

Leach MJ, Wiese M, Thakkar M, Agnew T (2018) Integrative health care – toward a common understanding: a mixed method study. Complement Ther Clin Pract 30:50–57. https://doi.org/10.1016/j.ctcp.2017.12.007

Lee I (2010) Ethnic differences in exercise and leisure time physical activity among midlife women. J Adv Nurs 66(4):814–827. https://doi.org/10.1111/j.1365-2648.2009.05242.x

Lee IM, Shiroma EJ, Lobelo F, Puska P, Blair SN, Katzmarzyk PT (2012) Effect of physical inactivity on major non-communicable diseases worldwide: an analysis of burden of disease and life expectancy. Lancet 380(9838):219–229. https://doi.org/10.1016/S0140-6736(12)61031-9

Mabry I, Young D, Cooper L, Meyers T, Joffe A, Duggan A (2003) Physical activity attitudes of African American and white adolescent girls. Ambul Pediatr 3(6):312–316

Martin M (2012) Surgeon general: don't let hair get in the way. NPR: National Public Radio.

Nelson TD, Benson ER, Jensen CD (2010) Negative attitudes toward physical activity: measurement and role in predicting physical activity levels among preadolescents. J Pediatr Psychol 35(1):89–98. https://doi.org/10.1093/jpepsy/jsp040

Parra-Medina D, Wilcox S, Salinas J, Addy C, Fore E, Poston M et al (2011) Results of the heart healthy and ethnically relevant lifestyle trial: a cardiovascular risk reduction intervention for African American women attending community health centers. Am J Public Health 101(10):1914–1921. https://doi.org/10.2105/AJPH.2011.300151

Pekmezi D, Ainsworth C, Desmond R, Pisu M, Williams V, Wang K et al (2018) Physical activity maintenance following home-based, individually tailored print interventions for African American women. Health Promot Pract:1524839918798819. https://doi.org/10.1177/1524839918798819

Poobalan AS, Aucott LS, Clarke A, Smith WCS (2012) Physical activity attitudes, intentions and behaviour among 18–25 year olds: a mixed method study. BMC Public Health 12(1):640. https://doi.org/10.1186/1471-2458-12-640

Reed M, Julion W, McNaughton D, Wilbur J (2017) Preferred intervention strategies to improve dietary and physical activity behaviors among African-American mothers and daughters. Public Health Nurs 34(5):461–471. https://doi.org/10.1111/phn.12339

Resnicow K, Baranowski T, Ahluwalia JS, Braithwaite RL (1999) Cultural sensitivity in public health: defined and demystified. Ethn Dis 9(1):10–21

Staffileno BADF, Minnick APF, Coke LADA-BC, Hollenberg SMMD (2007) Blood pressure responses to lifestyle physical activity among young, hypertension-prone African-American women. J Cardiovasc Nurs 22(2):107–117

The Barna Group (2008) New statistics on church attendance and avoidance. 3 Mar 2008

Thompson WM (2011) Physical inactivity of black adolescent girls: is it all about attitude? Home Health Care Manag Pract 23(3):186–192. https://doi.org/10.1177/1084822310390879

US Department of Health and Human Services (2010) Leading causes of death. Women's Health USA, USA

US Department of Health and Human Services (2018) In: Promotion ODPH (ed) Physical activity guidelines for Americans, 2nd edn. Office of Disease Prevention and Health Promotion, Washington, DC

Webb FJ, Khubchandani J, Hannah L, Doldren M, Stanford J (2016) The perceived and actual physical activity behaviors of African American women. J Community Health 41(2):368–375. https://doi.org/10.1007/s10900-015-0106-1

Wilbur J, Miller A, Fogg L, McDevitt J, Castro C, Schoeny M et al (2015) Randomized clinical trial of the women's lifestyle physical activity program for African-American women: 24- and 48-week outcomes. Am J Health Promot. https://doi.org/10.4278/ajhp.140502-QUAN-181

Williams WM, Alleyne R, Henley AT (2017) The root of physical inactivity among African-American women: identifying exercise friendly hairstyles. J Natl Black Nurses Assoc 28(2):26–31

World Health Organization (2014) Physical inactivity: a global public health problem. http://www.who.int/dietphysicalactivity/factsheet_inactivity/en/. Accessed 2 June 2014

Wellness and Integrative Health Strategies for Rural Populations

11

Lindsay Huse

11.1 Introduction

Nearly 20% of the US population lives in rural and frontier areas. Many of these populations have significant differences from urban populations that create disparities in how they experience disease and achieve health and wellness. Rural populations frequently struggle to access health care, both in terms of affordability and finding providers across the spectrum of care. Ratios of primary care providers, specialists, skilled care facilities, and home health care providers are typically higher than in urban areas. While public health nurses are frequently the main providers of some health services in underserved rural populations, capacity to continually see higher numbers of sicker patients is limited. Nurses in all specialties have an opportunity to apply an integrative health framework to improve the health of these populations in ways that are highly accessible, affordable, and build overall resiliency into population health.

Rural populations experience challenges in accessing nutrition, safe opportunities for physical activity, and encounter unique stressors that drive numerous acute and chronic disease conditions. However, they often possess cultural and traditional strengths that can be leveraged using an integrative framework to improve these areas. This chapter will define rural and frontier populations, explore rural population disparities, and discuss the strengths and challenges rural populations face in terms of health behaviors. It will apply an integrative nursing approach to assessing the health and wellness needs of rural populations, ensure inclusion of populations in determining their own needs and outcomes, and provide evidence-based, holistic wellness strategies that are both culturally- and patient-centered.

L. Huse (✉)
Public Health Nursing, Public Health Division, Wyoming Department of Health, Cheyenne, WY, USA
e-mail: lindsay.huse@wyo.gov

© Springer Nature Switzerland AG 2021
A. Vermeesch (ed.), *Integrative Health Nursing Interventions for Vulnerable Populations*, https://doi.org/10.1007/978-3-030-60043-3_11

11.2 Definition of Rural and Frontier Populations

Rural areas are defined by the U.S. Census Bureau as any area that is not urban; urban areas are characterized by larger populations over 50,000 people or may be a cluster of 2500–50,000 people living in close proximity. Approximately 19% of the population lives outside of these urban areas or clusters. The Federal Office of Rural Health Policy indicates a rural area as any outside of a metropolitan area, defined as over 50,000 people. By this slightly expanded definition, 18% of the US population is considered rural (Health Services and Resource Administration n.d.).

Rural populations experience significant differences in health outcomes when compared to their urban counterparts, such as higher rates of acute and chronic diseases, injury, and death. This poorer health and lower life expectancy is owed to numerous factors driven by rural geography. Large areas of isolation lead to the need for consistent, reliable transportation to manage increased travel times to access services. Fewer individuals living nearby mean fewer people able to provide services and jobs. Lack of employment leads to decreased socioeconomic status and inability to afford health care. Employers in rural areas are less likely to provide health insurance to their employees, and lower wages mean difficulty in purchasing it independently (Rural Health Information Hub n.d.-a). Additionally, rural populations engage more frequently in unhealthy behaviors. A 2013 study using the Behavior Risk Factor Surveillance System (BRFSS) highlighted that people living in rural areas had higher rates of smoking, drinking, poor sleep, overweight, and lower rates of participation in health behaviors (Matthews et al. 2017).

Populations living in rural areas also differ demographically. Veterans, including those with higher disability ratings, more commonly reside in rural geographies in the USA. Rural demographics can vary even more widely by state and county. Rural populations are more frequently male, living in poverty, over the age of 65, and may have lower education levels (Rural Health Information Hub n.d.-b).

Frontier areas exist in nearly every state; these areas are defined in numerous ways depending on agency and funding source. However, they are generally characterized by the need to travel long distances to find services, sparse settlement of estimated 6–11 people per square mile (National Center for Frontier Communities n.d.; National Rural Health Policy Association 2016), and in most states, are considered the most remote designation (National Rural Health Policy Association 2016). Many states that are characterized by wide swaths of frontier present geographical challenges that go beyond distance or sparse populations. For instance, in Alaska, it is not uncommon for health care providers to travel by small airplane to reach remote villages to provide care for populations. Wyoming's mountainous geography necessitates careful planning to minimize travel during the winter months, when mountain roads into deep frontier towns may become suddenly impassable. Not only is seeking out health care in such environments challenging, but choices taken for granted by more urban populations to live healthy lifestyles may not even be present for rural and frontier populations. Taken together, experiencing widely different determinants of health often leads to these populations suffering numerous disparities.

11.3 Disparities in Rural Populations

As previously noted, several challenges are present for those living in less populated areas of the USA. While the Affordable Care Act (ACA) was the first policy recognizing and making provisions for health care considerations at the frontier level, populations living in frontier areas still experience disparities in health due to access barriers and disparities inherent to rural populations in general.

Rural populations vary by race and ethnicity depending on location; for example, Black populations in the USA tend to live in metro areas, but in Mississippi and South Carolina they live more frequently in rural areas. Native American populations are frequently concentrated in rural areas near their tribal settlements, but in some states the rates are nearly even, such as in Idaho and Hawaii, and predominantly reside in metro areas in Massachusetts and Mississippi. Even within a state itself, there may be great variability in population characteristics between rural and metro areas (James et al. 2017). Adequate customization of integrative wellness strategies hinges on understanding the differences setting rural populations apart, including their challenges and strengths. BRFSS data compiled from 2012–2017 indicated that racial and ethnic health disparities exist within rural populations, even as rural populations themselves are considered a health disparity population. Rural Black, Hispanic, and American Indian/Alaska Native populations were more likely to rate their health as poor or fair in comparison to their White, Non-Hispanic counterparts. Likewise, these groups reported more days of physical and mental distress, and days of limited physical activity due to physical, mental, or emotional problems than Non-Hispanic Whites. However, rural Black populations were the least likely to report having never seen a physician and had the highest rates of having completed cervical and breast cancer screenings in the past 3 years, compared to other rural groups (James et al. 2017).

While race and ethnicity can signal disparities for health interventions, poverty is considered a major factor contributing to decreased health status, regardless of race. As previously discussed, populations living in rural areas may have lower educational attainment and fewer employment opportunities, leading to lower income status, lack of health insurance, and poor access to health care services (Rural Health Information Hub n.d.-a) and non-metro areas experience higher levels of poverty than metro areas. Poverty appears to be an even more significant driver of some health indicators than race. In one study, when adjusting for poverty, race, and neighborhood, poverty had a more significant impact on physical activity levels for both Blacks and Whites than either race or neighborhood (Hawes et al. 2019). Others found that while experiencing poverty individually increased both Blacks' and Whites' odds of having diabetes, *living* in a poor neighborhood increased the odds of having diabetes for all Blacks and poor Whites (Gaskin et al. 2014). Integrative wellness strategies will necessarily consider not only the individual circumstances and needs of the patient, but the environmental and community characteristics that drive those patients' behaviors and choices, or lack thereof.

11.4 Overview of Health Care and Wellness in Rural Areas

Rural and frontier populations frequently struggle with disparities based on race and location, and with a lack of access to health care across the spectrum. In the United States, the average number of medical doctors per 10,000 people in rural areas is 11. In metro areas, this rises to 31. Several states have as few as seven medical doctors per 10,000 people. Variability exists within the states as well, with some rural areas seeing as few as one medical doctor per 10,000. Rural areas have fewer practicing nurse practitioners and physician assistants per 10,000, despite efforts to fill rural gaps with such providers. While no agreed-upon ratio of providers-to-patients has been published, it stands to reason that populations that experience more frequent health care issues would benefit from easier access to health care providers. Indeed, better access to primary care providers would likely decrease some of the chronic negative health outcomes that come with living in rural areas. However, many primary care providers do not practice in rural communities due to lack of opportunities, lower patient insured rates, and poorer health care infrastructure (Rural Health Information Hub n.d.-b).

While major disparities exist in the ratios of primary health care providers between metro and rural/frontier areas, specialty care providers present an even more severe access challenge. Mental health providers are one of the greatest specialty care shortages in the USA. The Health Resources and Services Administration has indicated the entire nation as a national shortage area, with a few county-level exceptions (Rural Health Information Hub n.d.-b). Other specialists, such as orthopedists and cardiologists, are difficult to access for rural populations. Most specialists will opt to practice in more heavily populated locales that can support their practice, and support training and residency needs for aspiring specialists. Frequently this means that those living in rural populations will forgo specialist care, or will need to travel to the nearest city or even another state to seek care. Limited transportation options, affordability, lack of insurance coverage, and the time and effort to travel for care may present more of a challenge than some patients are able to overcome.

Rural populations in the USA are more frequently approaching the stage in life when more assistance with health care and daily living is necessary. While the median age of rural and frontier residents is just over 41 years of age, higher rates of older adults live rurally within over 20% of residents being over 65 years of age in some states (Rural Health Information Hub n.d.-b). With increased health care needs and a life expectancy of 77 years, many of these residents will need at least some level of care in their later years. Caregiving can be costly, leading many aging to rely on friends and family to assist them. As capacity for self-care and unskilled caregiving decreases, the need for skilled care becomes a necessity. An estimated 8% of rural counties have no post-acute skilled care facilities. While this is an improvement from the nearly 11% in 2008, it does indicate that there are still shortage areas for those in need of skilled care. Unaccounted for is the distribution of populations within counties and whether a county having a skilled nursing facility means that it is accessible. For instance, a large county with a population center may have facilities, but for rural aging populations on the other side of the county, transportation and cost may make access impossible (McMaughan et al. 2020).

Nursing home long-term care presents another challenge for aging rural residents as these facilities can be sparse, difficult in which to find a bed, and suffer from a shortage of skilled caregivers (Robert Wood Johnson Foundation n.d.). Additionally, long-term care in many rural areas is shifting to at-home or community-based care, meaning those who utilize facilities present more complex health challenges.

Public health departments and their nursing staff are excellent allies for the nurse planning integrative wellness strategies in rural and frontier areas. Public health nurses are competent in assessing population needs, have deep understanding of the drivers of health disparities in their communities, and are frequently extremely able to bridge communications and referrals within and across organizations. They work holistically to address the overall health of their populations while stewarding sparse resources and are a natural complement to nurses wishing to strategize integrative wellness plans for rural and frontier populations. Additionally, public health is often a central reference for rural populations seeking resources and even community resources. For instance, in Wyoming, local public health offices may be the most common point of comment for a newly pregnant woman to seek out presumptive Medicaid eligibility. As a nurse assists her with reviewing her eligibility, she may be referred into the Maternal Child Health home visitation program, and receive the phone number for the state tobacco quit line. As she is leaving, she may pick up a brochure for the nursing staff's Tai Chi for Better Balance class to give to her aging mother, who has arthritis and mobility issues and has been worried about helping her with a new baby. Additionally, she discovers while there that when the time comes, the local public health office is where she will need to take her baby for immunizations because the closest pediatrician is in the next county.

11.5   Integrative Nursing Approach to Rural Populations

The ability to assess the wellness needs of rural populations is necessary to tailor integrative approaches to the specific needs of these populations. Luckily, processes are already in place to assist nurses in gathering the kind of data necessary to determine these needs. Nearly every health department in the USA either conducts, or participates in, the assessment of community health and health needs. Based on the findings of these types of assessments, a community health improvement plan is typically put into place, with priority actions planned collaboratively across communities or health systems to address the greatest community needs. There are numerous frameworks for these assessments and plans, usually chosen based on resources, time, community engagement, and past frameworks. While individual patients may have a slightly different needs profile than the community at large, this is an excellent starting place, especially given that priority areas established under these assessments will have resources and commitments of effort behind them.

Participating in a community health assessment or needs assessment and subsequent improvement plan is a possible pathway for the integrative wellness nurse hoping to work with rural populations. These assessments are typically led by county health departments, or sometimes in concert with a hospital's needs assessment requirements under the ACA. These groups are consistently looking for individuals who are willing to participate in the process and a simple internet search for a county's community health assessment will usually yield documents with points of contact that can be used to initiate involvement. Health departments and hospitals can benefit from an integrative wellness lens being present on committees and workgroups as populations and interventions are considered.

If a county is not currently conducting an assessment, the most recent assessment and improvement plan can usually be found online, as these are public documents. Counties with significant rural and frontier areas will have looked closely at the health needs of these special populations, including primary and secondary data. If nurses are planning integrative care strategies and are not sure how to interpret the data included in these documents, the point of contact can usually put them in contact with a data analyst or manager who worked with the data originally.

Community health assessments and improvement plans are not the only means for assessing rural populations. Online tools such as countyhealthrankings.org (Robert Wood Johnson Foundation n.d.) list major health indicators and compare states and counties against each other and rank order them based on their performance on these indicators. This can be an incredible source of annually updated, secondary data. This tool may be more difficult to use in counties with both metropolitan and rural areas, so data should be considered carefully before using for decision-making.

An important reminder when planning any integrative wellness strategy, especially at a population level, is the concept of "Nothing about me without me," also known as true consensus, or more recently, shared decision-making. The concept creates a collaborative approach to decision-making about health interventions and choosing desired outcomes. The patient, or the population, is the driver of the decision with the health care (or public health) team considering the needs and values of the patient while providing input on options, potential outcomes, and resources. For instance, when assessing a rural population, perhaps the nurse identifies that a gap impacting the integrative health of the community is a lack of spiritual care. The nurse may feel that the absence of a local church building is the problem. However, had they included members of the population in discussing spiritual needs of the community, they may have instead identified that the gap exists with a very specific population in the community and that they prefer to meet in homes, or that the gap is being caused by something entirely different. Conversely, the nurse may discover that while spiritual care is important, a more urgent need expressed by the community is a lack of foot care clinics for a growing number of diabetics.

Inviting members of rural and frontier populations to participate in planning their own health not only decreases wasted time and resources, it builds trust and buy in. Integrative wellness is ultimately about holistic empowerment of a patient, or in this case, a population; this level of total care cannot be achieved without the participation and permission of the population being served.

11.6   Evidence-Based, Holistic Wellness Strategies

The most successful wellness strategies for rural populations will fit within the resource constraints of potentially vast and sometimes hostile geography, poverty, racial diversity, lack of access to care, and the values of the patient. Once the nurse has assessed their population, planning interventions should, when possible, be evidence-based and empower the patient. In this section, several integrative wellness strategies that are applicable to rural populations are discussed.

11.6.1 Meditation, Yoga, and Relaxation

Between 2012 and 2014, over 24% of rural and frontier residents were smokers (James et al. 2017). Tobacco use is the leading indicator of numerous adverse health outcomes, including lung cancer, heart disease, and chronic lung diseases. Health issues related to tobacco use cost the health care system over $330 million annually and cost many lives. Efforts to decrease tobacco use has been a longstanding goal of the public health and health care systems alike. Traditional clinical and public health methods to help patients quit have included both pharmacological and non-pharmacological methods (Centers for Disease Control and Prevention Center for Chronic Disease Prevention and Health Promotion 2019). The National Institute of Health Center for Complimentary and Integrative Health also reports successful tobacco cessation with the use of meditation, yoga, and relaxation techniques (National Institute of Health Center for Complimentary and Integrative Health 2017). The nurse planning integrative wellness strategies for tobacco cessation may consider designing a program that is comprised of traditional cessation methods and integrates meditation and mindfulness techniques either in part or as an entire package to improve quit rates with their patients. Collaborating with community yoga studios to offer special yoga classes for people attempting to quit tobacco may be another strategy. Other community resources that fit into an integrative approach may present themselves.

Meditation, yoga, and relaxation techniques have been successful techniques for individuals struggling with weight control (National Institute of Health Center for Complimentary and Integrative Health 2017). Given that overweight and obesity are major contributors to nearly every major negative health outcome from cancer to diabetes to heart disease and rural populations have higher rates of overweight and obesity, finding integrative strategies to help patients manage their weight is a high priority target. Traditional methods such as diet and exercise do not always address root issues of weight problems, which can range from stress and anxiety to mental health disorders and physiological imbalances. The exploration and integration of meditation and mindfulness or relaxation can address those variables ignored by traditional weight control methods. Yoga may have the added benefit of building physiological strength and flexibility and cardiovascular health while addressing stress and anxiety. Integration of such methods with healthy diet and exercise is likely to better address the entire constellation of causes within a patient and can be strategized into programs at the population level for greater impact.

Rural populations, including Veterans with high disability ratings and aging patients with conditions such as arthritis, benefit significantly from interventions that allow them to continue to function at their highest level, whether that means holding regular employment or simply being able to carry out activities of daily living. Additionally, given the opioid epidemic, the ability to help patients and special populations manage pain without the use of narcotic pain medications is even more important. Previously mentioned techniques such as meditation and relaxation can assist these rural populations with managing pain and limitations of movement. Additionally, integrative exercise techniques such as Tai Chi or yoga can maintain or restore range of motion, preserve musculoskeletal function, and improve pain levels. Some public health departments offer Tai Chi classes especially designed for preventing falls and improving arthritis symptoms in aging populations. The nurse planning integrative pain management for a special population such as one of these should consider ways to include as many tools for management of symptoms as possible.

Integrative wellness strategies are a natural fit for rural populations, who experience numerous disadvantages from racial and ethnic disparities to poverty and have fewer resources with which to address their needs. Rural and frontier residents may need treatment modalities that can be taught and self-managed at their homes in isolated geographies. Appropriate application of integrative strategies over time may decrease injuries and chronic diseases, which lessens the need to see providers frequently in areas that already experience provider shortages. Mentally and physically healthier populations are also better empowered to change their situations, whether that is seeking better employment or simply living longer on their own in their homes. In the end, the integrative wellness nurse best accomplishes this by including their patient, whether an individual or an entire community, in deciding what health—and getting there—will look like.

References

Centers for Disease Control and Prevention Center for Chronic Disease Prevention and Health Promotion (2019) Tobacco use. Available from https://www.cdc.gov/chronicdisease/resources/publications/factsheets/tobacco.htm#:~:text=CDC%E2%80%99s%20Response%20to%20Tobacco%20Use%201%20Help%20People,Risks%20of%20Tobacco%20Products%20for%20Young%20People.%20

Gaskin DJ, Thorpe RJ Jr, McGinty EE, Bower K, Rohde C, Young JH, LaVeist TA, Dubay L (2014) Disparities in diabetes: the nexus of race, poverty, and place. Am J Public Health 104(11):2147–2155. https://doi.org/10.2105/AJPH.2013.301420. PMID: 24228660; PMCID: PMC4021012

Hawes AM, Smith GS, McGinty E, Bell C, Bower K, LaVeist TA, Gaskin DJ, Thorpe RJ Jr (2019) Disentangling race, poverty, and place in disparities in physical activity. Int J Environ Res Public Health 16(7):1193. https://doi.org/10.3390/ijerph16071193. PMID: 30987098; PMCID: PMC6480690

Health Services and Resource Administration (n.d.) Defining rural population. Available from https://www.hrsa.gov/rural-health/about-us/definition/index.html

James CV, Moonesinghe R, Wilson-Frederick SM, Hall JE, Penman-Aguilar A, Bouye K (2017) Racial/ethnic health disparities among rural adults—United States, 2012–2015. MMWR Surveill Summ 66(SS-23):1–9. https://doi.org/10.15585/mmwr.ss6623a1

Matthews KA, Croft JB, Liu Y et al (2017) Health-related behaviors by urban-rural county classification—United States, 2013. MMWR Surveill Summ 66(SS-5):1–8. https://doi.org/10.15585/mmwr.ss6605a1

McMaughan D, Anikpo IO, Horel S, Ozmetin J (2020) Post-acute skilled nursing care availability in rural United States. Policy Brief. Southwest Rural Health Research Center. Available from https://www.srhrc.tamhsc.edu

National Center for Frontier Communities (n.d.) What is the frontier. Available from http://frontierus.org/what-is-frontier/

National Institute of Health Center for Complimentary and Integrative Health (2017) Tobacco cessation. Available from https://www.nccih.nih.gov/health/quitting-smoking

National Rural Health Policy Association (2016) Definition of frontier [Policy Brief]. Available from https://www.ruralhealthweb.org/getattachment/Advocate/Policy-Documents/NRHA FrontierDefPolicyPaperFeb2016.pdf.aspx

Robert Wood Johnson Foundation (n.d.) County health rankings. Available from https://www.countyhealthrankings.org/

Rural Health Information Hub (n.d.-a) Rural health disparities. Available from https://www.ruralhealthinfo.org/topics/rural-health-disparities

Rural Health Information Hub (n.d.-b) Rural data explorer. Available from https://www.ruralhealthinfo.org/data-explorer

Integrative Physical Activity Intervention Strategies and Influencing Factors for Latina Women

12

Amber Vermeesch

12.1 Introduction

The majority of Latinas are not engaging in recommended levels of physical activity (PA) and continue to be at increased risk for related health consequences compared to other populations (Guthold et al. 2018; National Center for Health Statistics 2018). The 2018 Physical Activity guidelines for adult Americans suggest that adults should participate in at least 150 min a week of moderate-intensity (e.g., brisk walking) or 75 min a week of vigorous-intensity (e.g., running or jogging) aerobic activity (U.S. Department of Health and Human Services 2018).

In 2018, National Center for Health Statistics (NCHS) (2020) fact sheet cited that 23.2% of US adults met the 2018 guidelines for PA engagement. In 2017, 18.9% of individuals identifying as Hispanic or Latino met the PA guidelines (National Center for Health Statistics 2018). PA is defined as physical exertion; exercise is a form of PA that is intentional in nature, usually repetitive, structured, and undertaken with the goal of improving health (U.S. Department of Health and Human Services 2018). The U.S Census defines Latinos as individuals of Latin-American descent (National Center for Health Statistics 2012). Latinos have reported less PA than Non-Hispanic Whites, and they have one of the highest prevalences of obesity compared to Non-Hispanic Whites (National Center for Health Statistics 2018, 2020). The prevalence of being overweight or obese is significantly different between racial/ethnic groups; it is lowest among Non-Hispanic Asian females (36.6%), followed by Non-Hispanic White females (64.6%), Hispanic females (78.8%), and Non-Hispanic Black females (80.6%) (CDC National Center for Health Statistics (NCHS) 2018). An increase or initiation of PA engagement could reduce negative health outcomes substantially.

A. Vermeesch (✉)
School of Nursing, University of Portland, Portland, OR, USA
e-mail: vermeesc@up.edu

© Springer Nature Switzerland AG 2021
A. Vermeesch (ed.), *Integrative Health Nursing Interventions for Vulnerable Populations*, https://doi.org/10.1007/978-3-030-60043-3_12

Motivation for PA appears to be related to changes in individual behavior. Researchers have found that increasing individuals' motivation, including Latinas, has successfully led to behavior change in a variety of health arenas including increased colorectal screening, increased medication adherence, substance abuse treatment, and improved diet (Wahab et al. 2008). Frederick et al. (1996) found that women who had an underlying intrinsic nature to their motivation to exercise were more likely to exercise, a finding confirmed by Murcia et al. (2007) among European Spanish women. Murcia et al. (2007) also found that Spanish women who were amotivated spent less time exercising. Cultural and demographic factors (e.g., acculturation, family obligations, number of children) as well as motivation type have been suggested as influencing participation in PA (Frederick et al. 1996; Vermeesch and Stommel 2014).

Strong evidence shows that insufficient physical activity shortens life expectancy and increases the risk of many adverse health conditions, including major non-communicable diseases such as coronary heart disease, type 2 diabetes, and breast and colon cancers (Lee et al. 2012). Additionally, Latina adults in the USA have a disproportionate health disparity compared to other populations related to increased burden of chronic disease due to low levels of PA engagement (Benitez et al. 2016). Because much of the world's population is inactive, this link presents a major public health issue.

Sustainable and successful interventions should be family-centered, social, and culturally tailored as well as derived from triangulating data from multi-method research. By analyzing multiple methods together from different types of collected data, triangulation leads to a broader understanding and increases the overall applicability of the data gathered. Interventions meeting these criteria are, by nature, integrative as they encompass multiple aspects of motivation to engage in physical activity.

An integrative health approach is one in which the client and the provider work together to facilitate healing and wellness using a variety of modalities and treats clients as whole persons (Kligler et al. 2015). Critical pieces of integrative health include the use of biomedical, sociocultural determinants of health, lifestyle, self-care, and partnership between client and provider, in pursuit of optimal health and wellness.

12.2   Intervention Strategies

Sufficient levels of exercise are associated with reduced risk for being overweight, developing diabetes mellitus, reduced risk of stroke, osteoporosis, and breast cancer and, therefore, individuals should engage in recommended levels of exercise to aid in achieving optimal health (Lee et al. 2012; Masterson Creber et al. 2017). According to Masterson Creber et al. (2017), Latinas who reported difficulty finding time to engage in physical activity were more likely to be obese. Exercise is an important, modifiable health behavior that is linked with reduction in stroke, obesity, and risk for developing weight-related illness such as diabetes mellitus (Larsen et al. 2017). This is a historic pattern that has endured and needs remedy.

12.2.1 Factors Associated with Exercise

Among Latinas, researchers conclude that acculturation, income, education, perceived health status, and number of children are related to exercise (Benitez et al. 2017; Tovar et al. 2018). The paragraphs below review literature on the relationship of each of these factors with exercise among Latinas.

For some Latinos, *curanderos*, or lay healers found predominately in the American Southwest, play an important role in healthcare and see themselves as important players in combating unhealthy changes in diet encountered by Latinos living in the United States. Clark et al. (2010) conducted focused interviews with *curanderos* who worked with Latinos of Mexican heritage to determine the *curanderos'* views of and beliefs regarding obesity causes, particularly in children, in Latino families. Clark et al. (2010) conducted 1 and 2 h interviews with seven *curanderos* and found that they attributed the rates of obesity, in part, to the change in foods eaten by Latinos and the decrease in breastfeeding resulting from a cultural shift away from more traditional beliefs that Latinos encountered while living in the United States. The *curanderos* viewed Anglo-centric interventions targeted for reducing obesity rates to be culturally alienating and provided the example of starting obesity reduction interventions too late, after the individuals are already obese, rather than earlier in life to prevent obesity. For example, they suggested culturally tailored obesity reduction interventions should start with pregnant women because pregnant women expect to be told what to do either from a healer or a doctor. This expectation of being told what to do could incorporate changes in diet and physical activity to help prevent obesity among Latinas.

By investigating and eventually incorporating the role of acculturation's effect on exercise among Latinas, perhaps interventions can be designed to break through the acculturation barrier and reach less acculturated Latinas and find ways to encourage exercise.

12.3 Motivation and Exercise

Motivation is an important factor that can be applied directly to increasing exercise among adults and is an important construct to focus on when investigating exercise in Latinas. In general, adult learners are more motivated to learn when they value the learning. The concept of valuing learning can be applied to Latinas in terms of tailoring interventions to increase exercise by incorporating family values since families are considered important (Berg et al. 2002; Lussier and Richard 2007; Sanders 2005). Eyler et al. (1998) conducted a series of focus groups with women from diverse backgrounds and found that among minority women, lack of motivation is a major barrier to exercise. Since individuals with extrinsic and intrinsic motivation tend to exercise more, determining types of exercise motivation is a worthy pursuit among minority women if interventions are to be designed to ultimately increase their participation in exercise. Frederick et al. (1996) found that women who had an underlying intrinsic nature to their motivation to exercise were more likely to exercise, a finding confirmed by Moreno et al. (2007) among European Spanish women. Moreno et al. (2007) also found that European Spanish women who were amotivated spent less time exercising. Moreno et al. (2007) conducted a cross-sectional study using a quantitative survey to collect data to validate the Behavioral Regulation in Exercise Questionnaire-2.

Regulation is the degree to which an individual has intention to engage in a certain behavior, in this case, physical activity (Markland and Tobin 2004). Individuals fall on a continuum of self-regulation ranging from amotivation to extrinsic and intrinsic regulation (Deci and Ryan 1985; Ryan and Deci 2000). Amotivation is completely non-self-determined, and individuals who are regulated by amotivation do not value the behavior. On the other end of the spectrum is intrinsic motivation where activities are engaged in for the pure enjoyment of the activity; intrinsic motivation is completely self-determined (Deci and Ryan 1985). At the middle of the spectrum is extrinsic regulation, where the individual focuses on goal-oriented achievement, i.e., a focus on rewards and punishments for engaging in the behavior.

According to the self-determination theory, individuals who have intrinsic motivation are more likely to engage in and continue to exercise than those with extrinsic motivation (Deci and Ryan 1985). Wilson and Rodgers (2004) concluded self-determination is a practical framework to study exercise motivation types among women. Determining exercise predictors and emphasizing intrinsic exercise motivation among Latinas that also incorporate potentially important cultural components is paramount in the design of sustainable and effective interventions to increase Latinas' exercise.

12.4 Triangulation

Triangulation is a method of analyzing data from multiple sources including qualitative and quantitative data to reduce limits of a one-dimensional view that may be present with using only one method. It allows researchers to combine methods to provide richer data that leads to a stronger understanding through multiple lenses of analyzing. The end data gathered from using triangulation methods can increase understanding and lead to a cohesive picture of the phenomena studied. The goal of using methodological triangulation is to glean information not available through the sole use of either quantitative or qualitative methods. With triangulation, researchers can extend findings beyond the quantitative goal of predictive causation relationships between variables, to a deeper description of the phenomena being studied (i.e., exercise motivators and barriers), not available any other way. With qualitative data, the participants provide rich data and a deeper sense of the women who are the participants in a study and insight into their exercise motivators and barriers. The origin of this method stems from the idea that combining methods can "enhance nurse researcher's efforts to describe and conceptualize the multifaceted complexity of the human response to illness and various healthcare situations" (Shih 1998). Otherwise, researchers risk, "Limiting data to only one data collection method limits insight" (Carter et al. 2014).

12.5 Implications for Nursing Practice, Education, and Research

From multiple studies, it is apparent that participants viewed exercise as a positive endeavor and value the results, both physical and mental, of exercise. Nurses should incorporate these positive attitudes and value of the benefits of exercise into their patient care. Understanding the changing views of Latinas as they become more acculturated to the United States is imperative if nurses and other healthcare workers are to effectively educate their patients regarding exercise as both a health promoting activity and a disease prevention strategy. In general, the more Americanized a Latina is, the more likely she is to report exercise as one of her daily activities. Nurses need to encourage more physical activities. This encouragement may take the form of designing and implementing culturally tailored interventions that incorporate preferred forms of exercise, such as dancing, with family-centered activities.

Latinas have some of the same barriers to exercise as other groups of women. They have competing obligations including going to work, caring for children, and doing housework; activities that leave little or no time for them to exercise. One of the keys to potentially effective interventions to engaging in exercise is to incorporate factors that help to alleviate their competing obligations such as integrating exercise more into their daily lives by providing childcare options for mothers who want to exercise or through education on how to increase exercise in the work settings. Another avenue might include drawing upon social support networks to help Latinas find others who are interested in exercising to enable them to motivate each other.

As healthcare providers, nurses are able to be more involved in the education of our patients regarding what exercise is and what "counts" as exercise. Exercise is Medicine (EIM), an initiative launched in 2007 by the American College of Sports Medicine, has many healthcare provider resources to call providers to action to assess and prescribe exercise and patient education of physical activity strategies (Sallis 2015). Targeting Latinas' perception of exercise is an important focus area for education as well as for practice. One example for patient education would be to educate patients that walking and working labor intensive jobs are forms of exercise. Smart device apps that count steps could be a way to share this information with patients. These potentially protective factors may be able to be harnessed through education to help Latinas feel good about their everyday incidental exercise and highlight their everyday exercise as something valuable and healthy. Additionally, healthcare providers can aid Latinas who are transitioning into American culture, to maintain behaviors that are protective of their health.

Understanding Latinas' perceptions of exercise can help to better guide practitioners to presenting exercise in a culturally sensitive manner. Through education by practitioners, Latinas may be more likely to report exercise if they are educated to think of some activities of daily living as exercise. Understanding the perceived effects of exercise such as improved general physical health, mental health, and physical aesthetics can help to guide future exercise interventions.

12.6 Conclusion

Nurses have a critical role in affecting interpersonal and cultural influences associated with increasing motivation to exercise for Latinas. The acculturation process and associated cultural aspects affecting exercise should be incorporated into future research and patient education. These strategies are in line with principles of the integrative nursing that emphasize the importance of person-centered and relationship-based healthcare strategies to optimize wellness (Kreitzer and Koithan 2014). PA education should incorporate extrinsic regulation among Latinas to maximize effectiveness. Additionally, social support and built environments such as neighborhood parks should be included (Munet-Vilaró et al. 2018; Murillo et al. 2020). Nurses are well poised to be on the front line of PA education and should be proactive in future PA interventions informed by integrative health approaches.

Acknowledgements The author would like to acknowledge the aid of research assistant, Gavin McBride, MS, Student of Physical Therapy, for assistance with literature review.

References

Benitez TJ, Dodgson JE, Coe K, Keller C (2016) Utility of acculturation in physical activity research in Latina adults: an integrative review of literature. Health Educ Behav 43(3):256–270. https://doi.org/10.1177/1090198115601042

Benitez TJ, Tasevska N, Indiana KC, Keller C (2017) Cultural relevance of the transtheoretical model in activity promotion: Mexican-American women's use of the process of change. J Health Dispar Res Pract 10(1):20–27

Berg JA, Cromwell SL, Arnett M (2002) Physical activity: perspectives of Mexican American and Anglo American midlife women. Health Care Women Int 23(8):894–904

Carter N, Bryant-Lukosius D, DiCenso A, Blythe J, Neville AJ (2014) The use of triangulation in qualitative research. Oncol Nurs Forum 41(5):545–547. https://doi.org/10.1188/14. ONF.545-547

Clark L, Bunik M, Johnson S (2010) Research opportunities with curanderos to address childhood overweight in Latino families. Qual Health Res 20(1):4–14. https://doi. org/10.1177/1049732309355285

Deci E, Ryan R (1985) Intrinsic motivation and self-determination in human behavior. Plenum, New York, NY

Eyler A, Baker E, Cromer L, King A, Brownson R, Dontalle R (1998) Physical activity and minority women: a qualitative study. Health Educ Behav 25:640–652. https://doi. org/10.1177/109019819802500510

Frederick C, Morrison C, Manning T (1996) Motivation to participate, exercise affect, and outcome behaviors toward physical activity. Percept Mot Skills 82:691–701

Guthold R, Stevens GA, Riley LM, Bull FC (2018) Worldwide trends in insufficient physical activity from 2001 to 2016: a pooled analysis of 358 population-based surveys with 1·9 million participants. Lancet Glob Health 6(10):e1077–e1086. https://doi.org/10.1016/S2214-109X(18)30357-7

Kligler B, Brooks AJ, Maizes V, Goldblatt E, Klatt M, Koithan MS, Kreitzer MJ, Lee JK, Lopez AM, Mcclafferty H, Rhode R (2015) Interprofessional competencies in integrative primary healthcare. Glob Adv Health Med 4(5):33–39

Kreitzer MJ, Koithan M (eds) (2014) Integrative nursing. Oxford Press, New York

Larsen B, Marcus B, Pekmezi D, Hartman S, Gilmer T (2017) A web-based physical activity intervention for Spanish-speaking Latinas: a costs and cost-effectiveness analysis. J Med Internet Res 19(2):e43. https://doi.org/10.2196/jmir.6257

Lee IM, Shiroma EJ, Lobelo F, Puska P, Blair SN, Katzmarzyk PT, Lancet Physical Activity Series Working Group (2012) Effect of physical inactivity on major non-communicable diseases worldwide: an analysis of burden of disease and life expectancy. Lancet 380(9838):219–229

Lussier M, Richard C (2007) The motivational interview in practice. Can Fam Physician 53:2117–2118

Markland D, Tobin V (2004) A modification to the behavioural regulation in exercise questionnaire to include an assessment of amotivation. J Sport Exerc Psychol 26(2):191–196

Masterson Creber RM, Fleck E, Liu J, Rothenberg G, Ryan B, Bakken S (2017) Identifying the complexity of multiple risk factors for obesity among urban Latinas. J Immigr Minor Health 19(2):275–284. https://doi.org/10.1007/s10903-016-0433-z

Moreno J, Cervello E, Martinez A (2007) Measuring self-determination motivation in a physical fitness setting: validation of the Behavioral Regulation in Exercise Questionnaire-2 (BREQ-2) in a Spanish sample. J Sports Med Phys Fitness 47(3):366–374

Munet-Vilaró F, Chase SM, Echeverria S (2018) Parks as social and cultural spaces among U.S.- and foreign-born Latinas. West J Nurs Res 40(10):1434–1451. https://doi.org/10.1177/0193945917692310

Murcia JAM, Gimeno EC, Camacho AM (2007) Measuring self-determination motivation in a physical fitness setting: validation of the Behavioral Regulation in Exercise Questionnaire-2 (BREQ-2) in a Spanish sample. J Sports Med Phys Fitness 47(3):366–374

Murillo R et al (2020) Frequency of seeing people walk and aerobic physical activity among Latino adults. J Phys Act Health 17(2):211–216

National Center for Health Statistics (2012) NCHS data on obesity. Retrieved from http://www.cdc.gov/nchs/data/factsheets/fact_sheet_obesity.pdf

National Center for Health Statists (2018) Health, United States, 2019 – data finder. CDC/National Center for Health Statistics/Division of Analysis and Epidemiology. https://www.cdc.gov/nchs/data/hus/2018/026.pdf

National Center for Health Statists (2020) NCHS data answering the nation's health questions. https://www.cdc.gov/nchs/about/factsheets/factsheet_nchs_data.htm

Ryan R, Deci E (2000) Self-determination theory and the facilitation of intrinsic motivation, social development, and well-being [Research Support, U.S. Gov't, P.H.S.]. Am Psychol 55(1):68–78

Sallis R (2015) Exercise is medicine: a call to action for physicians to assess and prescribe exercise. Phys Sportsmed 43(1):22–26. https://doi.org/10.1080/00913847.2015.1001938

Sanders M (2005) On the floor: excellence in teaching: adult learning strategies for motivation. ACSM's Health Fitness Journal 9(4):26–28

Shih FJ (1998) Triangulation in nursing research: issues of conceptual clarity and purpose. J Adv Nurs 28(3):631–641

Tovar M, Walker JL, Rew L (2018) Factors associated with physical activity in Latina women, a systematic review. West J Nurs Res

U.S. Department of Health and Human Services (2018) Physical activity guidelines for Americans, 2nd edn. U.S. Department of Health and Human Services, Washington, DC

Vermeesch AL, Stommel M (2014) Physical activity and acculturation among U.S. Latinas of childbearing age. West J Nurs Res 36(4):495–511. https://doi.org/10.1177/0193945913507341

Wahab S, Menon U, Szalacha L (2008) Motivational interviewing and colorectal cancer screening: a peek from the inside out. Patient Educ Couns 72(2):210–217

Wilson P, Rodgers W (2004) The relationship between perceived autonomy support, exercise regulations and behavioral intentions in women. Psychol Sport Exerc 5:229–242. https://doi.org/10.1016/S1469-0292(03)00003-7

Nursing Strategies to Reduce Perceived Stress Among Vulnerable Student Populations Preparing for NCLEX

13

Kaye Wilson-Anderson

13.1 Teaching Undergraduate Nursing Students: Holistic Reflective Approach

Nursing educators are charged to foster a safe and engaging learning environment and one that will facilitate graduate's success in nursing school and ultimately on the National Council Licensure Exam (NCLEX). Passing the NCLEX is required of all graduates from accredited baccalaureate or associate degree nursing program to become registered nurses prior to practice. While nurse educators desire to teach, and assist nursing students, they often feel very overwhelmed with increasing faculty shortage, class sizes, and escalating change in healthcare. The question arises, "how can nurse educators best address the needs of the learner"? This chapter will explore a variety of "best practices" focused on holistic reflective teaching approaches to ensure that nurse educators specifically have needed skills to meet diverse and vulnerable student populations.

As nurse educators, we teach our nursing students to implement "best practice" healthcare. This practice involves holistically assessing the client's physical, emotional, spiritual and environmental status (Wilson-Anderson 2020). This approach is a must because healthcare involves populations from diverse ethnic, cultural, language, economic and often complex social structural homes and communities. This same complexity is reflected in the nursing student population. Thus, it is imperative that nursing faculty approach each student's learning needs holistically. A holistic reflective teaching practice provides the nurse educator insights into how the student best learns, assist in identification of language challenges, impacting socio-economic concerns, ethnic, cultural context on learning and awareness of the student's support system. Additionally, this practice leads the student to reflect on

K. Wilson-Anderson (✉)
University of Portland, Portland, OR, USA
e-mail: wilsonb@up.edu

© Springer Nature Switzerland AG 2021
A. Vermeesch (ed.), *Integrative Health Nursing Interventions for Vulnerable Populations*, https://doi.org/10.1007/978-3-030-60043-3_13

their learning practices and how their personal background contributes to their ways of learning. Further, this approach leads students to examine integrative health modalities noted in the literature to be effective in assisting students to manage test anxiety, focus, and resilience.

13.2   Review of Literature

As early (2004) Duldt-Battey (2004) highlighted the need of nurse educators to incorporate the use of holistic educational practice to foster nursing student's success and in doing so, assisting the student in understanding the importance of approaching client care in a holistic manner. Duldt-Battey went on to state that "students in touch with their harmonious and whole selves are healthy, energetic, alert and self-motivated" (346). Further Duldt-Battey described the student that "experiencing holistic discord may exhibit anger, resentfulness, guilt, hopelessness, despair, self-doubt, and depression" (346).

Brock (2010) completed a quantitative study with 256 undergraduate business school students. The most reported step associated with transformative learning was *critical reflection*. The two next most reported steps were *disorienting dilemmas* and *trying on new roles*. The researcher used the findings of this study to provide additional validation of Mezirow's hypothesis on the significance of critical reflection to create changes in perception.

Vickous (2018) examined student identified variables that were deemed as supporting their success in nursing school and NCLEX. One of the first variables noted was that of "holistic support and encouragement from faculty" (49). Students emphasized that nursing faculty must seek to assess and understand students' external variables, the students' perception of these variables and adapt the nursing curriculum to ensure success of all students. Just as nurses utilize holistic assessment of clients to foster quality healthcare outcomes, nursing faculty should be compelled to do the same for nursing students to promote quality nursing education which will ultimately ensure "best healthcare outcomes."

Bernard (2018) noted that utilizing Mezirow (1996) transformative learning theory involving learner reflection, discussions and evaluation of their present lens of knowing, lead to the development of new expanding viewpoints. Based on Mezirow et al. (2000), the following ten steps that should be anticipated and shared with learners to promote full engagement of the transformative learning theory:

1. A disorienting dilemma
2. Self-examination with feelings of fear, anger, guilt, or shame
3. A critical assessment of assumptions
4. Recognition that one's discontent and the process of transformation are shared
5. Exploration of options for new roles, relationships, and actions
6. Planning a course of action
7. Acquiring knowledge and skills for implementing one's plans
8. Provisional trying of new roles

9. Building competence and self-confidence in new roles and relationships
10. A reintegration into one's life on the basis of conditions dictated by one's new perspective (p. 22)

Bice and Bramlett (2019) provided case studies as exemplars for clearly implementing Kolcaba's holistic comfort teaching strategy into nursing curriculum. Additionally, they go on to describe the use of Kolcaba's theory in enhancing the overall school of nursing environment to promote nursing faculty satisfaction and self-efficiency. Further, Goodwin et al. (2007) proposed that utilizing Kolcaba's holistic comfort theory in nursing education will lead to students experiencing, "true learning … in a lingering process of comfort that invites the opening of windows to a future of lifelong learning" (p. 286).

Moore (2017) clearly describes strategies to incorporate holistic teaching to assist freshman nursing students in beginning their nursing career. To provide exemplars and engage students, Moore incorporated storytelling from her practice. Students were led in a variety of activities utilizing the holistic approach to explore and examine a variety of nursing concepts and health needs and then to reflect on how these concepts and needs related to them personally. Moore reported a 90% student attendance for all classes with students engaging in verbal discussions and written reflections. Finally, students reported gaining focus and understanding of themselves and a drive to provide holistic nursing. This approach has often for the first time provided vulnerable student populations a space in which to examine external variables that cause them stress and incorporate learned integrative health modalities in addressing these needs (Mezirow et al. 2000; Wilson-Anderson 2020).

13.3   Implementations to Support Holistic Nursing Education

To ensure best nursing student NCLEX outcomes, this author has recognized the importance of approaching nursing students holistically and encouraging students in personal reflections. The magnitude of this educational strategy has become more apparent as senior nursing students have grown in their awareness of their strengths and areas that need strengthening to ensure success on their first NCLEX attempt following graduation. National Council for State Board (National Council of State Boards of Nursing 2019) data indicate that graduates that are not successful on their first NCLEX attempt are 50% more likely to not be successful on their second attempt. The significance of this achievement is beyond passing NCLEX but also maintaining the graduate's confidence, promoting financial security and facilitating achievement of future life goals.

Implementing a holistic personal assessment and plan to prepare for NCLEX leads students to focus on their nursing knowledge, testing skills, and exploration of any external variables that could potentially impact their NCLEX performance (Oregon Board of Nursing NCLEX Pass Rates n.d.). Further, students are encouraged to explore integrative health implementations such as mindfulness, exercise, and diet to address test anxiety, resilience, and life work balance (Wilson-Anderson

2020). Over the past 2 years, these strategies have demonstrated an increase in NCLEX pass rates above the national average for this baccalaureate nursing program (National Council of State Boards of Nursing 2019).

Further, graduates that were not successful on their first attempt, passed on their second attempt with 99–98% passing on their third attempt (Oregon State Board of Nursing 2019). In working, one on one, with graduates who were not successful, this author led students in reviewing their preparation time, as well as evaluating possible external variables that potentially impacted their success. Through this examination, it was discovered that most graduates had allowed an external variable to impact their testing performance. Graduates implemented a plan to deal with the identified external variable. External variables included: personal or family health concerns, ending significant relationships, relocating for their first nursing job and a need to address a past traumatic event or test anxiety. Once the graduate worked through the identified external variable, they found that focusing on the NCLEX testing experience became attainable (Wilson-Anderson 2020).

Beyond incorporating holistic reflective teaching in preparing nursing graduates for NCLEX success, this educator implements this educational strategy with all levels of nursing students. As the literature identified, the holistic reflective teaching strategy has facilitated an encompassing approach that fosters empowerment of students in strengthening study skills, addressing personal needs/challenges, and enhancing their self-efficiency. This educational approach provides faculty a framework to ensure that the ever-increasing diversity nursing student population are fostered and mentored in a positive learning environment and are successful in the nursing journey. Further, diversifying the nurse workforce is imperative to provide quality inclusive healthcare for the growing diverse population of America and the world (Oregon Board of Nursing NCLEX Pass Rates n.d.; Wilson-Anderson 2020).

13.4 Conclusion

As outlined in the review of literature, there are multiple academic reports of enhanced student learning outcomes utilizing holistic teaching strategies, holistic teaching based on Kolcaba's holistic comfort theory and the use of Mezirow's transformative learning theory which emphasizes reflection. Learners are directed in the identification of means to attain new roles, designing of a plan to achieve the new role and finally, development of empowerment to execute steps in gaining empowerment to achieve. Further, a plan to assist nursing graduates succeed on NCLEX utilizing a holistic reflective approach is presented.

The use of a holistic reflective teaching strategy promotes nurse educators in mentoring student nurses in a personal examination of holism and reflection. This teaching strategy facilitates students in moving through Mezirow's transformative learning theory and promotes student empowerment, self-efficacy and provides a framework for nurse student-faculty engagement to ensure student success. Finally, through utilizing holistic reflective practice, students gain a personal awareness of the importance of client-centered reflective holism approach when providing "quality nursing care" to ensure quality healthcare outcomes. Additionally, students gain personal knowledge of integrative health modalities that support management of stress, anxiety and foster resilience. Personal experience in utilizing these modalities increases students' confidence incorporating integrative health modalities into their nursing practice (Chinnery et al. 2019).

References

Bernard RO (2018) Nurse educators teaching through the lens of transformative learning theory: a case study. Doctoral dissertation. 10751211. ProQuest, Ann Arbor, MI

Bice AA, Bramlett T (2019) Teaching nurses from a holistic comfort perspective. Holist Nurs Pract 33:141–145

Brock SE (2010) Measure the importance of precursor steps to transformative learning. Adult Educ Q 60:122–142

Chinnery S, Appleton C, Marlowe JM (2019) Cultivating students' reflective capacity through group-based mindfulness instruction. Soc Work Groups 42(4):291–307. https://doi.org/10.1080/01609513.2019.1571760

Duldt-Battey BW (2004) Using the holistic paradigm in teaching. In: Oermann MH (ed) Annual review of nursing education. Springer Publishing Co., New York, NY, pp 345–355

Goodwin M, Sener I, Steiner SH (2007) A novel theory for nursing education. J Holist Nurs 25:278–284

Mezirow J, (1996). Beyond Freire and Habermas: Confusion. A response to Bruce Pietrykowski. Adult Education Quarterly. 46(4);237–239

Mezirow J et al (2000) Learning as transformation: critical perspectives on theory in progress. Jossey-Boss, San Francisco, CA

Moore AK (2017) Unflipping the classroom: introducing the values of holistic nursing at the freshman level. Am Holist Nurs Assoc 37:8–10

National Council of State Boards of Nursing (2019) NCLEX pass rates. https://www.ncsbn.org/Table_of_Pass_Rates_2019.htm

Oregon Board of Nursing NCLEX Pass Rates (n.d.). https://www.oregon.gov/osbn/Documents/Resource_passrates.pdf

Oregon State Board of Nursing (2019) Personal communication

Vickous SL (2018) Promoting undergraduate nursing student success in a small liberal-arts college. Doctoral dissertation. 10839456. ProQuest, Ann Arbor, MI

Wilson-Anderson K. (2020) NCLEX success. Nurs Pers. neponline.net

Complementary and Integrative Health Approaches for Women's Mental Health

Patricia Anne Kinser, Jo Lynne W. Robins, and Nancy Jallo

14.1 Introduction to General Complementary and Integrative Health Approaches

Approximately 33% of adults and 12% of children in the United States use complementary and integrative health approaches for promoting health and intervening with health problems (National Center for Health Statistics 2015). As the evidence grows to support the use of these approaches for health and wellness, healthcare professionals must be knowledgeable about complementary and integrative health approaches in order to provide patient-centered care. This knowledge will allow healthcare professionals to discuss these approaches with patients, to accommodate patients who choose to use them, and to be involved in the work of the many institutions that now provide complementary health approaches in an effort to provide integrative care to their patients. For example, many boards of nursing across the United States have approved certain complementary approaches as part of nursing scope of care, hence it is highly relevant that nurses enhance their knowledge in this field. In this chapter, we will review briefly the topic of complementary health approaches and integrative healthcare and provide exemplars of how these may be used for women's mental health.

It is essential for healthcare professionals to be aware of these general approaches and understand the key terms in the field before specifying their use for mental health. The term *complementary health* is used when describing interventions that are used along with and "complementary to" conventional medical interventions

P. A. Kinser (✉) · J. L. W. Robins · N. Jallo
Virginia Commonwealth University School of Nursing, Richmond, VA, USA
e-mail: kinserpa@vcu.edu; jwrobins@vcu.edu; njallo@vcu.edu

© Springer Nature Switzerland AG 2021
A. Vermeesch (ed.), *Integrative Health Nursing Interventions for Vulnerable Populations*, https://doi.org/10.1007/978-3-030-60043-3_14

(National Center for Complementary and Integrative Health 2020). Complementary approaches are typically wellness-focused and driven usually by an underlying holistic view of health, such that health is maintained through mental, social, spiritual, and physical balance (National Center for Complementary and Integrative Health 2020). *Conventional, or allopathic*, medicine is the dominant form of care delivery in the United States, with particular strength in addressing acute situations through biomedical, surgical, and pharmaceutical interventions (National Center for Complementary and Integrative Health 2020). The typical underlying belief system in conventional medicine is disease-focused, whereby that health is the absence of disease. However, patients and healthcare professionals have increasingly become aware of the limitations of conventional medicine to address chronic health conditions, patient symptoms, quality of life, and overall health and wellness (National Center for Complementary and Integrative Health 2020). *Integrative health* is a term used to describe the coordination of care such that conventional and complementary health approaches are used together in a thoughtful, planned way (National Center for Complementary and Integrative Health 2020). It is patient-centered, delivered by a team of biomedical, allied, and complementary health professionals working collaboratively and respectfully to deliver accessible, evidence-based, personalized, coordinated care with an emphasis on disease prevention and health, healing, and wellness promotion (Leach et al. 2018; Hilbers and Lewis 2013). The term *alternative health* is used when there is a practice that is used instead of conventional medical care. However, it is rare that people use only alternative approaches; as such, *alternative health* is not the focus of this chapter (National Center for Complementary and Integrative Health 2020).

It is well documented that health professionals require additional knowledge in this area. A survey published in 2018 of 1247 healthcare providers found that 82.5% agreed to a lack of complementary and integrative therapy knowledge and 65% indicated it was the patient who initiated the conversation (Aveni et al. 2018). Factors influencing health professional's familiarity, comfort, and use of integrative therapies included personal and clinical experience as demonstration of effectiveness (Aveni et al. 2018).

Scientific research on many complementary and integrative health approaches is ongoing, so information about safety and effectiveness may not be available for every approach. Further, historically, research in this area was not high quality. However, more and more well-designed studies are underway, particularly led by nurse scientists, and researchers are continually learning more about these approaches and the patients who might benefit the most from them. For example, in an integrative review of 101 complementary and integrative health therapies, Andrade and Portella (2017) found the evidence base is growing and methodological quality is continually improving. The suppositions and complexity of some of these therapies (e.g., acupuncture, Ayurvedic and Traditional Chinese Medicine) challenge current gold standard study designs, namely randomized, placebo controlled clinical trials. Future development of systematic reviews and meta-analyses is essential, as is the design of future research using comparative effectiveness and pragmatic trial design, all of which will foster translation of effective therapies into clinical practice.

Engagement in complementary and integrative health may provide positive experiences for both healthcare professionals and patients. Patients report increased satisfaction with care and empowerment in self-care through caring, supportive partnerships (Crocker et al. 2017; Foley and Steel 2017). In a synthesis of complementary and integrative health outcomes, Hilbers and Lewis (2013) found that incorporation of integrative therapies consistently increased patient satisfaction with care, filled gaps in treatment effectiveness (e.g., chronic, complex including chronic pain; desired alternative to pharmaceuticals; health promotion), and that communication and trust among integrative and allopathic providers increases referrals and enhanced safety. The following are important recommendations for healthcare professionals interested in engaging their patients in complementary and integrative health: (1) Be receptive to benefits and limitations; (2) Focus on patient-centered partnerships by asking about the use of and goals for integrative therapy as well as assessing patients' spiritual beliefs and needs; (3) Be as knowledgeable as possible to answer questions; and (4) Establish referral sources.

One easily accessible, up-to-date, and evidence-based resource is the National Institutes of Health's National Center for Complementary and Integrative Health (NCCIH) (http://nccih.nih.gov/). This resource is easily searchable and provides a variety of useful information as well as links to other trustworthy sources. The NCCIH provides a classification system for complementary approaches and integrative health into three categories: mind-body practices, natural products, or other. Table 14.1 provides a brief snapshot of the three categories and examples of each of them. One of the most reliable sources about use of complementary approaches in

Table 14.1 Categories of complementary health approaches and examples

Category of complementary approaches	Examples
Mind-body practices	• Yoga • Chiropractic or osteopathic manipulation • Meditation • Acupuncture • Relaxation techniques—guided imagery, breathing exercises, progressive muscle relaxation • Tai chi • Qi Gong • Hypnotherapy • Feldenkrais method • Alexander technique • Pilates • Rolfing structural integration • Trager psychophysical integration
Natural products	• Herbs/botanicals • Vitamins and minerals • Probiotics
Other	• Traditional healers • Ayurvedic medicine • Traditional Chinese medicine • Homeopathy • Naturopathy • Functional medicine

the USA is the National Center for Health Statistics (NCHS) National Health Interview Survey (NHIS), in which thousands of Americans are interviewed about their health- and illness-related experiences (National Center for Health Statistics 2015). In the most recent survey, the most commonly used approaches by US adults were natural products (~18%; most commonly fish oil), deep breathing exercises (~11%), yoga (~10%), chiropractic/osteopathic manipulation (~8%), meditation (~8%), and massage (~7%). The practice of yoga, tai chi, and qi gong has increased significantly since the prior survey in 2007. The 2012 report is available, along with a press release and graphics, at https://nccih.nih.gov/research/statistics/NHIS/2012.

The 2012 NHIS survey suggests that, generally, people choose complementary approaches as methods to maintain health and wellness or to relieve symptoms associated with an illness (National Center for Health Statistics 2015). For example, over 90% of individuals using yoga reported that they chose this approach for maintaining wellness, stating that they felt yoga helped motivate them for physical activity, enhance sleep, and manage stress. In addition, over a quarter (25%) of yoga practitioners stated they had stopped or significantly cut back on their use of substances such as cigarettes and alcohol (National Center for Health Statistics 2015). The health-related benefits of this and other complementary approaches warrant close attention for the health and wellness of the nation.

14.2 Exemplars of Complementary Health Approaches for Women's Mental Health

Given that the majority of users of complementary and integrative health approaches are women (National Center for Health Statistics 2015), it is relevant in this chapter to focus on three approaches commonly used by women for enhancing mental health: guided imagery, tai chi, and yoga. Research studies are beginning to reveal promising findings about the positive effects for promoting women's mental health and healthcare professionals are calling for these meditative mind-body approaches to be integrated into regular clinical practice (Innes et al. 2008; Hutson and McFarlane 2016). In a review of data from the 2012 NHIS survey, specific gender differences were identified: women were twice as likely to report use of meditative approaches and among the most frequently used were yoga and tai chi; more women than men found these practices to be more helpful for stress management (Upchurch and Johnson 2019). Three research studies conducted by the chapter authors are presented here to further inform the evidence on approaches, so that healthcare professionals may support and educate their patients in these therapies, and to foster engagement in future related research.

14.2.1 Tai Chi for Improving Mental Health in Women

Background: Tai chi is an ancient mind-body practice combining movement and breath to elicit the relaxation response. New evidence suggests that the particular movement and postures of tai chi result in improved psychological well-being (Osypiuk et al. 2018). Tai chi practice has been increasing over the last decade and its use transcends age, race and socioeconomic status as well as chronic health conditions (Hutson and McFarlane 2016; Wayne et al. 2017). There are hundreds of research studies on tai chi published in the literature. With regard to mental health outcomes relevant to women, Tong and colleagues conducted a systematic review of studies with findings to suggest that tai chi increases self-efficacy (Tong et al. 2018). A systematic review and meta-analysis found that tai chi improved depression, anxiety, and psychological well-being (Wang et al. 2013).

Brief description of study: In a randomized controlled mixed methods study, women ages 35–50 with a family history of cardiovascular disease were randomized to either the tai chi intervention or a wait-list control group. As reported by Robins et al. (2012a), this study tested the effects of a tai chi intervention that was designed to enhance stress management and improve immune and cardiovascular function. Integral to the intervention was a focus on educating participants about the meaning and purported physiological effects of the specific tai chi movements; further, the intervention involved discussions of spiritual beliefs, thoughts, and behaviors to foster application in daily life. The intervention had been tested previously in randomized clinical trials in individuals with human immunodeficiency infection (Robins et al. 2006), early stage breast cancer (Robins et al. 2013), and increased cardiovascular disease risk (Robins et al. 2016). In this study, participants randomized to the intervention group engaged in a weekly 60-min tai chi class for 8 weeks.

Summary of findings: A total of 63 women with increased waist circumference and a family history of CV disease participated in the study. The average age was 44 years; average body mass index was 32, and average waist circumference was 40 in. One quarter of the participants were African American and the remainder Caucasian. Qualitative data revealed the greatest challenge was finding time to practice outside of class but that they consistently remembered the meaning of the movements and it shifted their perceptions of stress and coping in daily life. Quantitative data analysis revealed significant decreases in fatigue, depression, and perceived stress over time in the tai chi group compared to the control group. Additionally, the tai chi group experienced significant increases in mindfulness, self-compassion, and spiritual thoughts and behaviors.

Clinical and research implications of the findings: Despite reporting minimal practice outside of a weekly 60-min class, the participants experienced lasting benefits in mental health 2 months post-intervention indicating tai chi may be an effective self-care strategy in women to improve mental health. This study contributes to a growing body of research evidencing the potential benefits of tai chi. Further, specific attention to study design and intervention delivery enhance the validity of the findings.

14.2.2 Guided Imagery for Improving Mental Health in Pregnant Women

Background: During pregnancy, maternal stress and the associated symptoms of anxiety, depressive symptoms, and fatigue have been associated with adverse pregnancy complications and negative birth outcomes (Ehrenthal 2016; Cardwell 2013). Pregnant African American women are especially vulnerable as they report high levels of psychological distress and increased susceptibility to the negative effects of these psychological stressors than other races/ethnicities (Noonan et al. 2016; Singh et al. 2017; Lu and Halfon 2003). While treatment options may exist, these vulnerable women may have concerns about pharmacological treatment effects and/ or limited financial resources to seek out non-pharmacological methods for symptom relief.

To address this need, our research team developed a 12-week guided imagery recorded intervention delivered on a compact disc player. Guided imagery is a mind-body therapy that is a dynamic psychophysiological modality which engages all of the senses to create a perception of an image with an emotional response linking the feeling state with the mind and body leading to a psychological or physiologic response (Menzies and Taylor 2004; Reed 2007; Achterberg 2002; Schaub and Burt 2013). The intervention incorporated components of relaxation focused breathing and a variety of multisensory guided images to promote reduction of stress, anxiety depressive symptoms and fatigue during pregnancy. Integral to the design of the intervention was multiple styles of imagery that focused on feelings and the desired end-state for pregnant participants, such as peace, calm, relaxed, and energized. This economical intervention was delivered via a device that could be integrated into their life and used at any time without concern for negative side effects, cost, or access.

Brief description of the study: As reported by Jallo et al. (2014, 2015), this longitudinal intervention study used a repeated measure mixed method design to test the effects of a guided imagery intervention on maternal stress, anxiety, depressive symptoms, and fatigue in pregnant African American women randomized to receive either the guided imagery intervention (intervention group) or to receive usual care (control group). The intervention group listened daily to the 12-week intervention and both groups were asked to record their daily stress levels.

Summary of findings: A total of 72 pregnant African American women participated in the 12-week study. The average age was 24.26 years, mean estimated gestational age at enrollment was 15.43 weeks, and the majority were not married, unemployed, and had a previous pregnancy. The participants completed measures at baseline, as well as 8 and 12 weeks. Quantitative data analysis indicated a reduction in daily stress scores and stress and anxiety scores at week 8 in the intervention group (Jallo et al. 2014). Qualitative findings indicated pregnant African American women lead stressful lives and they found the intervention to be beneficial to reduce stress and anxiety. They commented that the intervention offered a respite from their stressful lives, reduced the negative emotions stress responses, enhanced well-being and provided an opportunity to connect with their baby (Jallo et al. 2015).

Clinical and research implications of the findings: These findings suggest a guided imagery intervention may be effective in reducing perceived stress and anxiety and was perceived by the pregnant African American women as being beneficial in their stressful lives. This is a powerful finding as African American women potentially experience more stress with fewer resources (Guardino and Schetter 2014). Healthcare professionals can be reassured of the many benefits of the practice of guided imagery (Menzies and Jallo 2011). It requires nothing more than one's imagination, thus making it always available at no cost. This study provides preliminary evidence of acceptance, use, and effectiveness of guided imagery in pregnant African American women to manage stress and associated symptoms. Further study will build the evidence and support healthcare professionals to incorporate this stress management intervention as a necessary part of care for pregnant women to improve their health.

14.2.3 Yoga for Prenatal Depression

Background: At any given time in the United States, close to four million women are pregnant and, of these, nearly 20%, or 800,000 women, experience clinically significant depressive symptoms (Ashley et al. 2016; American College of Obstetricians and Gynecologists (ACOG) 2018). Depressive symptoms may include depressed mood, loss of interest, changes in weight, alterations in sleep, fatigue, guilt/ worthlessness, indecisiveness, and suicidality (American Psychiatric Association DSM-5 Task Force 2013). Despite that there are treatment options available, in the form of antidepressant medications and psychotherapy, many pregnant women have concerns with access to these treatments and/or concerns about side effects or adverse effects on their fetuses due to pharmacologic medications.

As such, research about complementary therapies for depressive symptoms during pregnancy is warranted. In an effort to address this need, our research team conducted a study to evaluate a self-management intervention entitled "Mindful Moms." This intervention involved three components: (a) a motivational interviewing-informed discussion between the research nurse and participant partnership about goal-setting for symptom management; (b) weekly instructor-led group prenatal yoga classes for 12 weeks; and (c) self-directed home-based physical activity consistent with individuals' goals. The intervention was built upon previous work that demonstrated women with depressive symptoms wish to actively engage in self-managing symptoms and view yoga as an accessible, gentle form of physical activity (Kinser et al. 2013; Kinser et al. 2012).

Brief description of study: As reported by Kinser et al. (2020), this longitudinal intervention study used a repeated measures design, coupled with qualitative methods, to evaluate the feasibility, acceptability, and preliminary effects of the "Mindful Moms" intervention for pregnant women with depressive symptoms. In this study, participants engaged in the intervention for 12 weeks during their pregnancy and received a follow-up visit at 6 weeks postpartum. Participants engaged in one-on-one interviews with the researchers at this 6 weeks postpartum visit.

Summary of findings: Forty-one women enrolled in the study, and a total of 27 women completed all aspects of the intervention and data collection. The average age of enrolled participants was 29.1 (5.3), with a mean estimated gestational age at enrollment of 17.5 weeks (5.6). The majority of participants were either married or cohabitating with a partner (76%), self-identified as black/African American (63%), and worked either part- or full-time (66%). The participants completed measures at baseline, mid-way through the intervention, at the end of the intervention, and again in the postpartum period (6 weeks postpartum). Quantitative data analysis indicated a reduction in depressive symptom, stress, and anxiety scores over time throughout the 12 weeks intervention, with sustained effects into the early postpartum period. Qualitative findings from the one-on-one interviews suggested that women who engaged in "Mindful Moms" gained a sense of empowerment for managing their depressive symptoms. They reported the importance of having an embodied experience of self-care and relief of symptoms, of sharing experiences in a safe space with other pregnant depressed women, and of receiving non-judgmental motivation and support from the study staff (Russell et al. 2020).

Clinical and research implications of the findings: These findings suggest that "Mindful Moms" appears to be a feasible and acceptable approach to enhancing self-management of depressive symptoms in pregnant women. Healthcare professionals working with pregnant women should be aware of the potential benefit of strategies such as mindful physical activity for helping women manage their depressive symptoms. However, because this was a small study that lacked an active concurrent control group, further large-scale research is warranted to evaluate fully the potential efficacy and effectiveness of such an intervention for pregnant women with depressive symptoms.

14.3 Conclusion

Complementary and integrative health approaches are inherently patient-centered and based on collaborative partnerships between patients and providers. However, before these approaches can be fully integrated into patient care, evidence from research studies is required to inform treatment decisions. Healthcare professionals should maintain and/or increase awareness that an evidence-based practice model combines the best research findings, clinical expertise, and patient values and preferences. The methodological quality of the evidence regarding meditative mind-body approaches is improving and methods for further strengthening it are ongoing (Kinser and Robins 2013; Kinser et al. 2016; Robins et al. 2012b). We have sought to contribute to healthcare professionals' expertise in this chapter, particularly in the area of yoga, tai chi, and guided imagery, which are generally safe and increasingly accessible complementary approaches for self-care and management of stress and depression in women. A key focus in each of these studies was intervention fidelity, to ensure that the intervention was delivered as designed to promote validity of the findings and translation to practice (Robins et al. 2018).

Given calls for integrative approaches to address mental health by reducing iatrogenic effects of pharmacologic treatments and enhancing improved outcomes (Lake and Turner 2017), it is timely and important for healthcare professionals gain comfort with discussing complementary and integrative health approaches with their patients.

References

Achterberg J (2002) Imagery in healing: shamanisms and modern medicine. Shambhala Publication, Inc., Boston, MA

American College of Obstetricians and Gynecologists (ACOG) (2018) ACOG Committee Opinion No. 757: screening for perinatal depression. Obstet Gynecol 132(5):e208–e212

American Psychiatric Association DSM-5 Task Force (2013) Diagnostic and statistical manual of mental disorders: DSM-5™, 5th edn. American Psychiatric Publishing, Inc., Arlington, VA

Andrade, Portella (2017) Research methods in complementary and alternative medicine: an integrative review. J Integr Med 16:6–13

Ashley JM, Harper BD, Arms-Chavez CJ, LoBello SG (2016) Estimated prevalence of antenatal depression in the US population. Arch Womens Ment Health 19(2):395–400

Aveni E, Bauer B, Ramelet A-S, Decosterd I, Ballabeni P, Bonvin E, Rodondi P-Y (2018) Healthcare professionals' sources of knowledge of complementary medicine in an academic center. PLoS One 12(9):e0184979

Cardwell MS (2013) Stress: pregnancy considerations. Obstet Gynecol Surv 68(2):119–129

Crocker RL, Grizzle AJ, Hurwitz JT, Rehfeld RA, Abraham I, Horwitz R, Weil A, Maizes V (2017) Integrative medicine primary care: assessing the practice model thorugh patients' experiences. BMC Complement Altern Med 17:490–497

Ehrenthal DB (2016) Preventive effects of birth outcomes: buffering impact of maternal stress, depression, and anxiety. Matern Child Health J 20:56–65

Foley H, Steel A (2017) Patient perceptions of clinical care in complementary medicine: a systematic review of the consultation experience. Patient Educ Couns 100:212–223

Guardino CM, Schetter CD (2014) Coping during pregnancy: a systematic review and recommendations. Health Psychol Rev 8(1):70–94

Hilbers, Lewis (2013) Complementary health therapies: moving towards an integrated health model. Collegian 20:51–60

Hutson P, McFarlane B (2016) Health benefits of tai chi: what is the evidence? Can Fam Physician 62:861–890

Innes KE, Selfe TK, Taylor AG (2008) Menopause, the metabolic syndrome, and mind body therapies. Menopause 15:1005–1013

Jallo N, Ruiz RJ, Elswick RK, French E (2014) Guided imagery for stress and symptom management in pregnant African American women. Evid Based Complement Alternat Med 2014:840923

Jallo N, Sayler J, Ruiz RJ, French E (2015) Perceptions of guided imagery for stress management in pregnant African American women. Arch Psychiatr Nurs 29:249–254

Kinser P, Robins J (2013) Control group design: enhancing rigor in research of mind-body therapies for depression. Evid Based Complement Alternat Med 2013:1–10

Kinser P, Goehler L, Taylor A (2012) How might yoga help depression? A neurobiological perspective. Explore (NY) 8(2):118–126

Kinser P, Bourguignon C, Taylor AG, Steeves R (2013) "A feeling of connectedness": perspectives on a gentle yoga intervention for women with major depression. Issues Ment Health Nurs 34(6):402–411

Kinser P, Robins J, Masho S (2016) Self-administered mind-body practices for reducing health disparities: an interprofessional opinion and call to action. Evid Based Complement Alternat Med 2016:2156969

Kinser P, Moyer S, Mazzeo S, York T, Amstadter A, Thacker L, Starkweather A (2020) Protocol for pilot study on self-management of depressive symptoms in pregnancy. Nurs Res 69(1):82–88

Lake J, Turner MS (2017) Urgent need for improved mental health care and a more collaborative model of care. Perm J 21:17-024

Leach et al (2018) Integrative health care-toward a common understanding: a mixed methods study. Complement Ther Clin Pract 30:50–57

Lu MC, Halfon N (2003) Racial and ethnic disparities in birth outcomes: a life course perspective. Matern Child Health J 7(1):13–30

Menzies V, Jallo N (2011) Guided imagery as a treatment option for fatigue: a literature review. J Holist Nurs 29(4):279–286

Menzies V, Taylor A (2004) The idea of imagination: an analysis of "imagery". Adv Mind Body Med 20(2):4–10

National Center for Complementary and Integrative Health (2020) Complementary, alternative, or integrative health: What's in a Name? Available from: https://www.nccih.nih.gov/health/complementary-alternative-or-integrative-health-whats-in-a-name

National Center for Health Statistics (2015) Trends in the use of complementary health approaches among adults: United States, 2002–2012. National health statistics reports; no. 79. National Center for Health Statistics, Hyattsville, MD. Available from: https://www.cdc.gov/nchs/data/nhsr/nhsr079.pdf

Noonan AS, Velasco-Mondragon E, Wagner FA (2016) Improving the health of African American in the USA: an overdue opportunity for social justice. Public Health Rev (37):12

Osypiuk K, Thompson E, Wayne PM (2018) Can tai chi and qigong postures shape our mood? Toward an embodied cognition framework for mind-body research. Front Hum Neurosci 12:174

Reed T (2007) Imagery in the clinical setting: a tool for healing. Nurs Clin North Am 42(2):261–277

Robins J, McCain N, Gray P, Elswick R, Walter J, McDade E (2006) Research on psychoneuro-immunology: tai chi as a stress management approach for individuals with HIV disease. Appl Nurs Res 19:2–9

Robins J, Elswick RK, McCain NL (2012a) Evolution of a unique tai chi intervention. J Holist Nurs 30:134–146

Robins J, Elswick RK, McCain NL (2012b) The story of the evolution of a unique tai chi form: origins, philosophy, and research. J Holist Nurs 30:134–146

Robins J, McCain NL, Elswick RK, Walter J, Gray DP, Tuck I (2013) Psychoneuroimmunology-based stress management during adjuvant chemotherapy for early breast cancer. Evid Based Complement Alternat Med 2013:1–7

Robins J, Elwsick RK, Sturgill J, McCain NL (2016) The effects of tai chi on cardiovascular risk in women. Am J Health Promot 30:613–622

Robins J, Jallo N, Kinser P (2018) Treatment fidelity in mind-body interventions. J Holist Nurs 37(2):189–199

Russell N, Aubry C, Rider A, Mazzeo S, Kinser P (2020) Mindful Moms: Motivation to self-manage depression symptoms. MCN, Am J Matern Child Nurs 45(4):233–239. https://doi.org/10.1097/NMC.0000000000000625

Schaub B, Burt M (2013) Imagery. In: Dossey B, Keegan L (eds) Holistic nursing. Jones &Bartlett, Burlington, MA, pp 363–396

Singh GK, Daus GP, Allender M, Ramey CT, Martin EK, Perry C, De Los Reyes AA, Vedamuthu IP (2017) Social determinants of health in the United States: addressing major health inequality trends for the nation, 1935–2016. Int J MCH AIDS 6(2):139–164

Tong Y, Chai L, Lei S, Liu M, Yang L (2018) Effects of tai chi on self-efficacy: a systematic review. Evid Based Complement Alternat Med 2018:1701372

Upchurch DM, Johnson PJ (2019) Gender differences in prevalence, patterns, purposes, and perceived benefits of meditation practices in the United States. J Womens Health 28:135–142

Wang F, Lee E-KO, Wu T, Benson H, Fricchione G, Wang W, Yeung AS (2013) The effects of tai chi on depression, anxiety, and psychological well-being: a systematic review and meta-analysis. Int Soc Behav Med 21(4):605–617

Wayne PM, Gagnon MM, Macklin EA, Travison TG, Manor B, Lachman M, Thomas CP, Lipsitz LA (2017) The mind body wellness in supportive Housing*MiWish* study: design and rationale of a cluster randomized controlled trial of tai chi in senior housing. Contemp Clin Trials 60:96–104

Integrative Strategies for American Indians

15

Michelle Kahn-John

Preamble: In my role as a nurse and Native American (NA) traditional wisdom keeper, it has always been natural for me to integrate as many pathways and approaches to wellness when caring for or coaching others about health and wellness. As I began to write this chapter, I experienced apprehension because this chapter focuses on strategies of integrative healthcare for American Indians (AI). I will discuss what is known about integrative health in AI communities, but the reason for my apprehension is much of this chapter is centered on historical experiences and the integration of Traditional Medicine/Healing (TM/H) alongside mainstream healthcare delivery systems. The invitation to write this chapter is an honor and see it as an opportunity to protect, advocate for and promote greater access to traditional healing and medicine for AIs while sharing insights about AI TM/H. I am a member of the Navajo Nation and my clans are as follows: I am Tótsohnii (Big Water) [maternal]), born for the Bit'ahnii (Folded Arms people) [paternal], and the Granddaughter to the TséŃjííkiní (cliff dweller, among the rocks, honeycombed rock dweller) [maternal as well as paternal grandfathers]. My upbringing was immersed in traditional Diné teachings, ceremonies, and exposure to rich cultural practices, language, and lifeways. My mom had an important role in our community and she spent much of her lifework praying for others, hosting ceremonies, preparing and administering herbal remedies but most importantly, she was a listener, an encourager, and a person with generous amounts of time, love and compassion for others. Though I have authentic insight, knowledge, and experience about AI TM/H, most of my experience is with my own community, the Diné Nation and my intertribal knowledge on TM/H is growing; however, remains limited. A consistent theme across all AI communities is that we must protect our cultural wisdom especially sacred knowledge and wisdom. I have been reminded frequently by my elders of how our indigenous knowledge and ceremony are to be protected and sharing of this sacred knowledge, especially with those outside of our culture has always been strongly prohibited. I chose to offer this work as a means to preserve and protect AI sacred cultural knowledge while creating opportunities for younger AI generations and healthcare providers to learn about respectful integrative healthcare strategies when working with AIs. Privacy and specifics about AI TM/H will remain protected as I instead offer key aspects and strategies for respectful integrative approaches when working with AI communities. I ask for grace from my AI relatives as I share this work with a good heart and with intent for health and wellness for all. Ahéhee (Thank You), Michelle Kahn-John, member of the Diné Nation.

M. Kahn-John (✉)
College of Nursing, University of Arizona, Tucson, AZ, USA
e-mail: mkahnjohn@email.arizona.edu

15.1   Introduction

This chapter on Integrative Strategies for American Indians (AI) will offer insights on the historical events experienced by AIs, demonstrate AIs had pre-existing culturally based and complex health systems, discuss historical events and the United States treaty-based healthcare delivery systems in AI communities, introduce exemplars of integrative health approaches in AI communities and highlight some strategies on ways to integrate culturally sensitive, complementary and traditional medicine and healing (TM/H) practices in AI communities. Much caution is taken throughout the chapter to maintain respect and protect the privacy of AI communities and their ancient healthcare systems, specifically the protected procedural and spiritual aspects of AI TM/H.

15.2   American Indian Health Disparity and Inequity

The current health of 5.2 million AI/ANs reflects inequity and disparity. These health inequities have existed for several centuries and coincide with the arrival of colonialist settlers. AIs experience disproportionate rates of chronic illness such as cardiac disease, cancer, unintentional injuries, diabetes, liver disease, mental illness, suicide and substance abuse (Adakai et al. 2018; United States Department of Health and Human Health Services 2020a, United States Department of Health and Human Services 2020). In 2017, the IHS per capita personal healthcare expenditure comparison reported expenditures of $4078 for AIs compared to $9726 for the US general population (United States Department of Health and Human Health Services 2020a). The poor social conditions and economic disadvantages in AI communities contribute to the disproportionate burden of chronic illness, decreased life expectancy, and decreased quality of life. Higher death rates among AI/ANs are attributed to liver disease, diabetes, unintentional injuries, suicide, homicide and respiratory disease. Solutions for chronic AI health disparity and inequity include increased funding and the development and implementation of AI/AN led culturally relevant, innovative and tailored integrative healthcare delivery models and interventions.

15.3   Complementary, Traditional, Indigenous
Health Approaches

The National Center for Complementary Alternative and Integrative Health (NCCAIH) indicates approximately 30% of the US population utilizes some form of complementary or alternative health approach (United States Department of Health and Human Health Services 2020b). Complementary health approaches are those used in addition to mainstream health approaches while alternative approaches are those used in place of mainstream approaches. The NCCAIH acknowledges integrative approaches as those that are holistic, patient-centered and inclusive of interventions that address the whole, including mental, emotional, functional, spiritual, social, and community aspects of health and wellness. Integrative approaches are coordinated and intentional efforts of HC providers, systems, organizations, and institutions that make these holistic approaches accessible to patients and communities. AI TM/H approaches and wellness practices delivered by "traditional healers" are considered "complementary," per the CCAIH definition.

The World Health Organization (WHO) defines Traditional Medicine (TM) and/or indigenous traditional medicine as "the sum total of knowledge and practices, whether explicable or not, used in diagnosing, preventing or eliminating physical, mental or social diseases. This knowledge or practice may rely exclusively on past experience and observation handed down orally or in writing from generation to generation. These practices are native to the country in which they are practiced. The majority of traditional medicine has been practiced at the primary health care level" (World Health Organization 2019). The WHO recognizes Traditional and Complementary Medicine (T&CM) as a global mainstay of healthcare delivery. The intent of the WHO T&CM 2014–2023 Strategy is to support development of innovative, safe, regulated, integrated infrastructure and approaches that create and increase access to T&CM by individuals, healthcare providers (HCP), healthcare systems (HCS), organizations, institutions, and governments who recognize T&CM as a "vibrant and expanding part of healthcare" (World Health Organization 2013). The specific objectives of the WHO T&CM 2014–2013 Strategic Plan is: (1) building the knowledge base and formulating national policies; (2) strengthening safety, quality, and effectiveness through regulation; and, (3) promoting universal health coverage by integrating T&CM services and self-healthcare into national health systems (World Health Organization 2019). Indigenous traditional medicine is now recognized by national and global healthcare agencies such as the NCCAIH, Indian Health Services (IHS), and the WHO, thus validating the importance of TM/H, T&CM as critical aspects of health delivery for AI populations.

15.4 Pre-existing American Indian Health Systems

Every society on the globe has distinct innate culturally informed health systems and wellness practices tailored to the unique needs of each population. Each population has distinct health systems that align with the geographical regions in which the population lives, and the climates associated with those regions. American Indians (AI), also referred to as Native Americans (NA), Alaska Natives (AN) hereafter referred to as AI, have occupied North American well before European and Spanish colonization. Each distinct AI tribal community has meaningful origin stories. From the AI worldview, health sustaining cultural knowledge, complex and holistic health systems and wellness practices are inseparable from the cosmic order of the universe. AI health and wellness systems are inseparable from spiritual beliefs and emphasize the importance of respecting, sustaining, and honoring relationships with all of nature and the universe. This awareness of and high regard for the interconnectedness and interdependence (relationships) among humans, nature, animals, spirits, and the Creator instilled beliefs, natural laws and obligations which serve as the foundation for health systems and practices in AI communities (Coyhis and Simonelli 2005; Kahn-John 2010; Grandbois and Sanders 2009). AI health and wellness systems and practices continue to exist today despite external efforts of colonization to eradicate AI culture, language, spiritual and ceremonial practices, and pre-existing health systems (Brave Heart and DeBruyn 1998; Whitbeck et al. 2004; Goodkind et al. 2012; Hartmann and Gone 2014; Cohen 1998).

AI health systems exist with a worldview that recognizes the sacredness of a shared consciousness between all animate and inanimate universal beings. This shared consciousness mandates respectful and interdependent relationships between humans, spirits, animals, nature, and a reciprocal obligation to acknowledge and care for beings and elements of the earth and universe. This awareness and high regard for a shared consciousness and existence is common amongst indigenous cultures. It is through the worldview and awareness of a profound shared consciousness that AI stories, teachings, moral and ethical principles which embody health sustaining and restorative knowledge systems and practices emerge. Begay and Maryboy (2000) elaborate on this AI worldview and offer this exemplar, the Navajo worldview is "naturally dynamic and everything evolves from a spiritual and cultural way of life rooted in the cosmic order" (p. 499). AI obligation to and reverance for this relationship with the universe is based on their understanding that intentional as well as unintentional human acts of disruption to this cosmic order are believed to bring harm, imbalance, disharmony, or illness.

Examples of human acts of disruption to the cosmic order may include bringing harm to or killing a living being, destruction of the earth or elements of the earth, and disrespect and disregard for the sometimes dangerous nature of natural elements and occurrences (e.g., earth, fire, air water, lightning, radiation, heat, cold). Illness, disease, and imbalance in the physical, mental, emotional and spiritual dimensions are believed to be brought on by acts of disruption to the cosmic order. These disruptions are believed to be transgenerational, impacting those directly perpetrating or experiencing the disruption as well as those connected through family lineage (children, grandchildren). For examples, in the Navajo culture, there are strict protective rules to be observed by expectant parents during pregnancy. The traditional teachings about pregnancy recommend the avoidance of witnessing or engaging in negative or destructive behaviors or occurrences. Parents are prohibited from hunting or witnessing traumatic events. These protective teachings provide a safe and nurturing prenatal environment for the developing fetus. Expectant parents are encouraged to seek out beautiful activities and environments, stay physically active, eat healthy, and get adequate rest to promote a healthy pregnancy and birth and also to establish a safe physical, psychological and spiritual environment for the birth of a healthy new baby.

The basis for teachings that guard against the witnessing of traumatic events demonstrates AIs were/are attuned with the post-traumatic mental and emotional sequelae that we now know as post-traumatic stress, acute stress disorder and historical trauma. Physical, mental, emotional, and spiritual health afflictions are believed to also emerge from ancestral traumatic events and physical or emotional afflictions from these events have the ability to transfer across generations. For example, a TM practitioner may explain to an AI patient who is seeking TM healing that their illness is related to an event that a parent or grandparent experienced or witnessed. This AI cultural inherent knowledge may be comparable to discoveries in genetic (e.g., transferability of genetic traits among family members) or epigenetic research and warrants further scientific exploration.

The entire pre-birth, life and death process has significant rites of passage commemorated by ceremony or celebration. It is during these important phases of life that health teachings are affirmed. An example is the adolescent ceremonies that mark the transition between childhood and adulthood. Many of the teachings and guidance offered during an adolescent coming of age ceremony in AI communities are about the importance of healthy eating, physical activity, developing strong moral and ethical character, and the strengthening of spiritual practices. Emphasis on diet, physical conditioning, spiritual practices, and moral and ethical responsibilities are all aspects of health promotion that have always been present in AI communities.

Symptoms of physical illness and psychological distress are known to result from exposure to trauma, loss, and grief. Distinct AI ceremonial and healing interventions are intended to purify, cleanse, and restore health, harmony, and balance to an individual or a family who has experienced trauma. Often these ceremonial interventions prescribed for grief, trauma, and loss are communal and call for the participation of family and community. Shared and collective healing interventions remind an individual of how much they are valued, loved, and supported. A unique feature of TM/H is the obligation and willingness by family and community to be present to assist during times of healing. The presence of family and community is believed to allow for collective sharing of the ceremonial interventional healing benefits. The patient receives therapeutic benefits of a healing intervention while family and other participants realize how they too become recipients of the shared therapeutic TM/H intervention.

The complex and integrative journey towards wholeness, health, and wellbeing begins pre-birth and continues throughout life. There is a constant awareness and recognition of the complex whole and the validation, attention, and balance that an individual must maintain in their physical, mental, emotional, spiritual realms while being constantly aware of the interactions and the obligation to sustain holistic health and wellness at each encounter with a living being or universal element.

Many of the principles of AI health, wellness, and ceremonial interventions overlap and revolve around a constant synthesis of spiritual practices. Spirituality is inseparable and remains the core of health and wellness interventions in AI communities. Behaviors that convey respect and reverence are foundational attributes for maintaining AI health, wellness, and spiritual practices. All is sacred and therefore, all acts including thoughts, speech, and behaviors must recognize the sacredness of entirety when journeying through life.

AI philosophies comprehend that wellness is actually a constantly moving point on a health-illness continuum. This continuum reflects the points between opposite extremes of dichotomous variables such as all points between health and illness, balance and imbalance, and harmony and disharmony. AI communities share the perception that illness, disharmony, and states of imbalance are the result of disruption to the natural cosmic order. AI teachings reflect the understanding of a mandatory interdependence amongst all living beings in the universe. All aspects of the universe are believed to have a consciousness, an awareness and a spirit and therefore must be acknowledged in our everyday thoughts, speech and behaviors. The AI worldview conceptualizes the depth and the interdependent nature of the universe and all within, then realizes the responsibility each of us has, as conscious human beings to not only tend to our personal human needs, but also the importance of acknowledging, protecting, respecting, and caring for the entire Universe as an equally important aspect of universal wellness. AI wisdom keepers understand dichotomous continuums exist and the constant shifts experienced on this continuum are relevant to all within the universe. The teachings further emphasize that everything in the universe has the potential to promote or diminish health. For example, elements such as fire, water, air, and earth are highly respected in AI culture. Each element has the power to sustain or diminish life. Too much water could cause a human, plant, or an animal to drown while too little water could induce dehydration and death. The same example can be applied to the recognition of both the necessity of and caution that must be extended to elements of air, oxygen, minerals, sunlight, darkness, temperature changes, and nutrition. Every exposure, ingestion, or interaction among universal life forms [living beings] and elements must occur with utmost awareness as well as cautious respect to maintain health and safety. Recognition of the impact of positive and negative interactions between humans, natural elements and universal life forms and how the quality of these interactions can either diminsih, sustain or promote health of self and others is central to AI culture and traditional AI health systems. Acts of respect and extensions of high regard to all living beings, elements, animals, nature, and the entire universe is highly prioritized in AI culture and core to the AI teachings, TM and existing health systems because each interaction between living beings and natural elements has the capacity to become both a dangerous life threatening affliction and/or a nurturing life giving resource.

AI health systems have always integrated complex philosophical understandings with spiritual beliefs, thereby recognizing the sacredness of all within the Universe. AIs synthesize and integrate spirituality, culture, health, and wellness practices alongside mainstream healthcare systems and approaches with a goal to move towards mental, emotional, spiritual and physical health and wellbeing. These ancient AI integrative practices inform the development of contemporary synergistic momentum driven by a mix of historical events, culture, traditional AI philosophy, innovation, and recognition of the importance of meaningful integrative wellness approaches.

Though TM/H can be much to complex to define, an evolving definition of TM/H gleaned from the input of (AI) traditional healers/practitioners (TH/Ps) who participated in two national meetings on TM is presented. "TM/H is the interrelational therapeutic processes involved in the application of sacred, mysterious, and spiritually informed AI/indigenous cultural knowledge systems and healing practices that are passed down from one generation to the next. TM/H is used to diagnose and treat physical, spiritual, mental, and emotional imbalances that result in illness and distress" (Esposito and Kahn-John 2020; National Institutes of Health Tribal Health Research Office (NIH THRO) 2019; Moorehead Jr. et al. 2015; Struthers et al. 2004).

TM/H practices are specific to each AI Nation and include brief (couple hours) as well as more extensive ceremonies (spanning multiple days). Because of the vast diversity as AI/AN tribal nations, communities, villages, and pueblos, it is difficult to discuss actual TM/H interventions without risking inaccuracy, ethical violations or cultural disrespect. For those interested in understanding more in depth aspects of TM/H further research and exploration can be sought in emerging publications within scientific literature that provide insights on AI tribe-specific TM/H interventions. To gain authentic knowledge about TM/H practices, I encourage those interested to respectfully request a time to speak directly to TM/H practitioners to engage in dialogue about the topic in a traditional AI manner while understanding and acknowledging that some topics remain private and can only be known by TM/H practitioners. Following traditional AI etiquette is highly recommended when seeking sacred knowledge and may require a traditional or spiritual gift offering. Therefore, it would be appropriate to seek guidance from local AI cultural experts on appropriate and culturally sensitive ways to seek this knowledge. Mentioned in the preamble to this chapter, protection of the sacred nature of AI TM/H practices will be maintained, therefore only a brief introduction and very general and superficial overview of select AI TM/H practice categories is discussed.

AI TM/H practitioners possess a broad range of cultural knowledge on traditional medicine and healing interventions. This knowledge can be organized into the following TM/H categories: diagnostics, purification and cleansing, and restoration of wellness, balance and harmony. Diagnostics involve a process to detect or diagnose the source of illness along with recommendations on ways to restore health and balance. Purification and cleansing interventions are intended to cleanse the body, mind, spirit, or a physical environment such as a home or building of negatie experiences, energies, illness or traumatic events. The interventions intended to restore wellness, balance and harmony vary widely and may include herbal remedies, prayers, chants, and ceremony. A few AI wellness models are shared to highlight philosophical underpinnings of AI TM/H and cultural health restorative practices.

Primordial AI health and wellness models acknowledge the importance and inclusion of the physical, mental, emotional, spiritual, and social dimensions of health and wellness. An integrative AI wellness model developed by an AI nurse scientist provides an exemplar of shared intertribal philosophies that sustain and promote health and wellness.

The Hózhó Wellness Model stresses the importance of the inclusion of AI cultural knowledge in healthcare delivery. Kahn-John, a member of the Diné Nation suggests the integration of mainstream healthcare practices alongside culturally relevant teachings found within the Diné (Navajo) Hózhó Wellness Philosophy may empower Diné with enhanced capacity to maintain physical, emotional, mental, spiritual, social and environmental health and wellness. Hózhó is a state of happiness, balance, health, beauty, harmony and embodies all that is positive and life sustaining. The Hózhó philosophy places ownership and responsibility on individuals to realize and integrate the philosophical teachings as a means towards sustaining health, happiness, harmony, balance, and wellbeing. The Hózhó teachings underscore the sacredness of life, and the responsibility of the Diyin Nohookáá

Dine'é (precious and holy earth-surface people—human beings) to be mindful and intentional with thoughts, speech, actions, and behaviors as we each journey towards health and wellness with awareness of the value of not only our own health, but also the health and wellbeing of others, and all beings within the entire universe. Conceptual attributes of the Hózhó philosophy include respect, relationships, thinking, reciprocity, discipline, positivity, love, happiness, and spirituality. Practice of the Hózhó attributes are believed by the Diné to assist in moving towards, sustaining, and perhaps achieving the revered state of Hózho.

15.5   American Indian Use of Traditional Medicine and Healing

AI health and wellness seeking behaviors are influenced by culture, levels of acculturation, economic status, healthcare access, access to traditional AI teachings and healing interventions and a multitude of psychosocial impacts of colonization. AIs may have strong preferential health seeking behaviors and may select TM/H as a sole approach to pursuing health or an integrative approach that integrates various health delivery approaches or complementary models.

The NCCAIH report AIs and Caucasians as the highest users of complementary approaches (United States Department of Health and Human Health Services 2020b). Kim and Kwok (1998) reported approximately 38% of AIs utilize TM/H interventions on a regular basis. It is unknown exactly how many AIs utilize TM/H, but evidence has demonstrated significant use patterns ranging between 38% upwards to 55% (Kim and Kwok 1998; Novins et al. 2004). AIs seeking healthcare in mainstream healthcare systems recognize the gaps in mainstream HC delivery models and cite they that lack spiritual, social, and environmental health considerations. Of interest is a study with Caucasian participants who utilized complementary health approaches. The participants cited reasons for preferring complementary approaches included dissatisfaction with mainstream HC approaches, effectiveness of complementary approaches, holistic focus, relationship focused care interventions, and personal journey (Heafner and Buchanan 2016). Several studies with AI populations demonstrate similar findings including the importance of a nurturing relationship between patient and healthcare provider or TM/H practitioner, cultural preference, and the desire to achieve transformative and holistic wellness in the realms of physical, mental, spiritual, emotional, social, and environmental health (Begay and Maryboy 2000; Joe et al. 2016a; Moghaddam et al. 2015). Further exploration of AI usage rates, perceptions and reasons behind preferences or avoidance of TM/H interventions would offer valuable insights that will surely contribute greater understanding of the significance of TM/H approaches in AI communities.

In mainstream and complementary health service approaches, there are regulating agencies and educational requirements to confirm authenticity and verify standardized training of all practitioners. The authenticity of Traditional Medicine Healers/ Practitioners (TMH/P) has historically occurred through the organic process of confirmation by a TMH/P mentor, family, and the tribal community. A fully ordained and/

or accomplished TMH/P often possess extensive cultural knowledge as well as practice knowledge on herbal gathering, preparation, and administration. Practitioners spend years learning ceremony, ritual, songs, chants, prayers, spiritual communication, interpretation of spiritual messages, and are expected to adhere to mandates of respect for all of nature and all living beings.

15.6 Authenticity of Traditional Medicine Healers/ Practitioners

On the Navajo Nation, groups of AI medicine practitioners, healers, and spiritual leaders formalized several traditional spiritual organizations as early as the 1970s to protect and promote traditional medicine, cultural knowledge, and healing and ceremonial practices. These organizations commenced for political reasons to defend and stop the desecration of AI cultural, spiritual, and ceremonial paraphernalia and practices. Over time, the organizations have served to provide AI expert cultural consultation for research initiatives and through their certifying processes have opened doors for TM/H practitioners to have TM skills acknowledged, accepted and integrated through employment opportunities in healthcare and educational settings. The three AI spiritual organizations on the Navajo Nation, the Diné Hataałii Association (DHA), Azee Bee Nahaghaa of Dine Nation Inc. (ABNDN), and the Diné Medicine Man's Association (DMMA) developed certifying processes, similar to board certifying practices found in medicine, nursing and in complementary practices (Azee Bee Nahgha of Dine Nation Inc. Azee Bee Nahgha of Dine Nation Inc. 2020; Navajo CARES Act 2020; Begaye 2017). Certification with one of these AI healing and spiritual organizations demonstrates commitment to protect AI ceremonial knowledge and spiritual practices while offering a non-traditional authentication process that verifies authenticity, by ordained TMH/Ps, for those seeking certification. From a cultural and traditional AI perspective, certification for TM/H practitioners is a non-traditional process and has been contentious. A benefit of the certifying process, though non-traditional, is that it provides data on the number of TM/H practitioners, their specialty practice category and offers a mechanism to verify authentic practice and encourage standards of authentic, safe and ethical practice. Authenticity of TM/H practices has become of great concern in AI communities because of the growing number of native and non-native practitioners who falsely claim knowledge and expertise in TM/H practices (Donovan 1997), further justifying the need for and benefit of a AI led and culturally sensitive regulating process or organizations that provide leadership, expertise and verification of authenticity for AI TM/H practitioners and their interventions.

These spiritual and ceremonial organizations on the Navajo Nation have become an essential and significant resource for those seeking AI cultural expert opinion on matters related to AI spirituality, ceremony, healing and cultural knowledge and practices. Indian Country (a term used by AI communities referring to the broad intertribal collective United States AI population) is often responding to a steady flow of researchers, private corporations, and healthcare organizations who have good intent, but perhaps lack important cultural insights which may then increase their risk for imposing ethical or cultural violations that may damage AI communties. For this reason, it is important that each AI community have a reserve of accessible and authentic cultural experts who can deliberate and offer valid expert cultural recommendations or guidance on how to navigate matters that pose a threat to the AI community. An important function of these spiritual and ceremonial organizations is to review research proposals, extend cultural expertise and serve as gatekeepers by offering, approvals, recommendations and sometimes objections to researcher proposals or proposed AI TM/H interventions that intend to promote health for AIs through the study or implementation of highly revered and protected AI cultural, spiritual, and ceremonial practices.

An introduction to the philosophical underpinnings of AI health systems and wellness practices has been presented. In the next section, a discussion is presented on how pre-existing AI healthcare systems were intended to be replaced with United States treaty-based mainstream healthcare services. Some mainstream health services for AIs continue to be managed by the United States Federal Government through the Indian Health Services and more recently are increasingly being managed by AI tribal Nations.

15.7   Treaty-Based American Indian Healthcare

The Indian Health Services (IHS) was established through the United States (US) Federal Government in 1787 based on Article 1, Section 8 of the US Constitution as a treaty obligation for the purpose of ensuring that comprehensive healthcare is available to citizens of federally recognized tribal nations (United States Department of Health and Human Health Services 2020c). The healthcare services were initially delivered by the U.S. Department of Defense, the same department that was at war with AI Nations, and services were eventually transitioned, managed and delivered by the IHS.

There are currently 574 federally recognized tribes in the US and IHS funds health services for 170 tribal, urban, and federal AI serving healthcare facilities across the nation (United States Department of Health and Human Health Services 2020a, United States Department of Health and Human Services 2020). The IHS cites the following as their mission, vision, and goals (United States Department of Health and Human Services 2020), Mission: to raise the physical, mental, social, and spiritual health of American Indians and Alaska Natives to the highest level, Vision: healthy communities and quality healthcare systems through strong partnerships and culturally responsive practices. The IHS goals are:

- to ensure that comprehensive, culturally appropriate personal and public health services are available and accessible to American Indian and Alaska Native people,
- to promote excellence and quality through innovation of the Indian health system into an optimally performing organization,
- to strengthen IHS program management and operations.

As noted in the mission and vision statements, the IHS recognizes the importance of culturally responsive practices which included spiritual health, as part of the comprehensive healthcare delivery system. In 1994, in a special IHS General Memorandum, Captain Michael Trujillo, the Director of the IHS signed to policy, support for the integration of traditional AI healing practices and ceremonies across federally funded IHS clinics and hospitals. The policy resulted in the development of the Traditional Cultural Advocacy Program (TCAP), through which Dr. Trujillo affirmed his commitment to protect and preserve rights of AI/ANs by advocating for the need to include TM/H practices in IHS settings. This policy encouraged the development of integrative exemplars of care that brought TM/H approaches within the walls of federally funded IHS, tribal and urban clinics as well as behavioral and hospital settings. This was a historic and meaningful feat for AI communities. Presented next is history on relevant and important US political milestones that contributed to development of integrative healthcare systems across Indian Country. A few exemplars of integrative healthcare settings will be shared.

Another relevant and historical milestone for AIs was when President Jimmy Carter signed the American Indian Religious Freedom Act (AIRFA) on August 11, 1978 (American Indian Religous Freedom Act CFR 1978; American Indian Religous Freedom Act 1996). The AIRFC declared "it shall be the policy of the United States to protect and preserve for American Indians their inherent right of freedom to believe, express and exercise the traditional religions of the American Indian, including but not limited to access to sites, use and possession of sacred objects and freedom to worship through ceremonials and traditional rites." Because the act was a joint resolution with congress, it was lacking provisions for enforcement. Enforcement was not achieved until another act was passed in 1993 which advocated for AIs to retain their sacred sites. In 1994, another amendment to the act allowed for legal use and transport of Peyote for the purpose of AI ceremony. A critique of the American Indian Religious Freedom Act is the use of the term "religion" which creates a misperception that AI ceremonial practices, use of sacred objects, and freedom to worship through ceremonies and rites are religious practices. AIs have clearly expressed their worldviews, beliefs, culture, spiritual practices, healthcare systems as ways of life and do not categorize these worldviews, beliefs or ways of life as religion. Health sustaining teachings, practices, and the use of ceremony in AI communities are inseparable from broader teachings that guide traditional AI worldviews. These two significant events led to the development of federal policies that opened doors, and once again made it permissible to openly practice and begin to develop culturaly aligned integrative systems of healthcare delivery for AIs.

The Southcentral Foundation (SCF) in Alaska, established in 1997 under the leadership of Rita Blumenstein and Lisa Dulchok is a premier exemplar of AI/AN health system integration. The SCF was successful in sustaining an integrated healthcare delivery model inclusive of Western mainstream medicine and Alaska Native (AN) medicine and healing approaches (Southcentral Foundation 2020). SCF employs Alaska Native healers, to facilitate talking circles, traditional counseling, and traditional physical modalities which encompass a form of traditional AN massage and healing touch. A traditional AN healing garden is available at the SCF Traditional Clinic to share wisdom on the sacred and therapeutic healing benefits of local native plant life. Tribal, urban, and IHS clinics and hospital settings across the nation followed suit and various tribe and community specific integrative models exist across Indian Country.

The Fort Defiance Indian Hospital (FDIH), now known as Tséhotsooí Medical Center (TMC) was successful in bridging inpatient psychiatric services with Diné

(Navajo) traditional healing interventions by employing male and female Diné traditional practitioners/healers and included them in the multidisciplinary treatment team comprised also of physicians, nurses, psychologists, therapist, social workers, behavioral technicians, special education teachers, and art therapists. This integrative model was the result of focus groups held within the community of Fort Defiance, AZ, on the Navajo Nation. Community-based focus groups insisted on integrating Diné cultural teachings and use of TM/H if the hospital intended on establishing an inpatient psychiatric facility for AI adolescents. The implementation team was successful in building an integrative model which contributed to the formal establishment of the Traditional and Cultural Services Department at the Fort Defiance I.H.S. Hospital in 2005. The TCS team offers accessible TM/H interventions to all AI community members. Traditional structures such as a Hogan and sweatlodge were built on site, within hospital grounds to ensure authentic and culturally aligned delivery of TM/H services.

The Chinle Comprehensive Healthcare Facility (CCHCF), an IHS hospital established an Office of Native Medicine (ONM) in 2000. The ONM, another exemplar of an integrated model in an AI community continues to offer patient-centered care and has a team of Diné Native Medicine practitioners that practice in a multidisciplinary team alongside western healthcare practitioners (Joe et al. 2016a, b). The ONM team has provided leadership in publishing literature which highligh the value and benefits of their integrated care services. This model of care offered by the Chinle ONM delivers culturally safe and competent care resulting in improved health equity and improved quality of care.

Despite the success of these AI integrative exemplars of integrated healthcare delivery, there have been some elements of concern regarding the practicality as well as the cultural safety and ethics associated with these models. There is a lack of funding and third-party reimbursement to support these complementary TM/H interventions. We run the risk of disrespecting the sacred when we bring sacred ancient AI practices into a mainstream healthcare settings. Therefore, careful consideration of the importance of cultural sensitivity and protection of the sacred is urged when implementing AI TM/H models. There may be instances where it is outright inappropriate to bring a sacred intervention into a mainstream setting or healthcare facility so culturally informed advisory groups (members of the AI/AN tribes, nations, bands, villages, and pueblos) must be part of the planning, implementation, delivery, approval and oversight of these integrated TM/H models.

15.8 Strategies and Consideration for Integrating Traditional American Medicine and Healing

It is important to consider all stakeholders when considering changes in the healthcare setting or the mechanisms of healthcare delivery. A few key stakeholders in successful integration of AI TM/H interventions are patients and family members, AI cultural experts, AI TM/H practitioners, healthcare administrators (HCA), healthcare funding agencies, and healthcare providers (HCP).

The delivery of mainstream healthcare interventions relies on implementation of evidence-based practice standards and interventions. The challenge for HCPs when considering safe integration of mainstream HC interventions alongside TM/H interventions is based on the requirement to deliver safe, evidence-based healthcare and despite the growing evidence to support the benefits of TM/H models and interventions, the evidence remains scarce. Discussions, culturally congruent research led by AI scientists and access to experts or educational resources can provide insights to safe integration of TM/H interventions and are recommended to assist in filling the current gap on TM/H interventions. Quality education and training on TM/H serves to inform mainstream HCPs while assisting them to become culturally aligned with the population they serve, thereby minimizing concerns they may have about the safety of integrative TM/H practices. Health Science Academic Institutions (nursing, medicine, pharmacy) must be supported and encouraged to develop curriculum on culturally safe, sensitive, aligned and congruent integrative approaches for an increasingly diverse population. Health science professionals are encouraged to expand practice knowledge by exploring and learning about TM/H practices, and the benefits of implementing culturally informed health intervention strategies. Cross-cultural educational exchanges for key stakeholders have the greatest capacity to promote collaborative, culturally aligned development of integrative systems of healthcare for AIs (Redvers et al. 2020; Struthers et al. 2004; Moss et al. 2005; Struthers et al. 2005; Struthers and Littlejohn 1999).

15.9 Conclusion

Significant advances are being made at the local, state, national, and global levels to transform healthcare delivery to include TM/H interventions for indigenous populations. A key message to all stakeholders as we embark on developing more effective integrative healthcare strategies for our diverse population is to expand practice knowledge beyond healthcare delivery systems and practices that rely solely on evidence-based research outcomes that may be inappropriately and/or overly focused on measures of intervention efficacy (Waldram 2013). Instead, a recommendation for all disciplines of healthcare providers and healers is to remain open to considering alternative ways of knowing, indigenous ways of knowing, and the benefits of inclusion of ancient transformative indigenous and AI healthcare systems and models that stimulate and uphold self-efficacy, transform, empower, and restore individual and collective culturally meaningful health outcomes. The Cultural Wisdom Declaration (CWD) inspired by a Tohono O'odham traditional AI elder, Mr. Chester Antone reminds us that AI TM/H practices belong to the AI/ANs and indigenous communities and do not require validation, permission, approval or compliance with regulations based on mainstream healthcare delivery systems (Antone et al. 2016). A culturally aligned approach, an AI approach with conscious intentionality designed for AI/AN communities is required as organizations such as the IHS, WHO, NCCIH, states, tribal nations, and local healthcare organizations partner to create healthcare delivery systems adapted to the unique needs of AIs and indigenous populations. With trust, respect, support, acceptance, and commitment as outlined in the CWD, we have the capacity to transform healthcare and significantly enhance the health and wellbeing of AIs and indigenous communities across the globe.

References

Adakai M, Sandoval-Rosario M, Xu F, Aseret-Manygoats T, Allison M, Greenlund KJ et al (2018) Health disparities among American Indians/Alaska natives – Arizona, 2017. MMWR Morb Mortal Wkly Rep 67(47):1314–1318

American Indian Religous Freedom Act Amendments of 1994 CFR (1996)

American Indian Religous Freedom Act CFR (1978). Available from: https://uscode.house.gov/statviewer.htm?volume=92&page=469

Antone C, Flores M, Kahn-John M, Solomon TA (2016) Cultural wisdom declaration. Substance Abuse and Mental Health Service Administration

Azee Bee Nahgha of Dine Nation Inc. Azee Bee Nahgha of Dine Nation Inc. (2020) Website of the ABNDN. Available from: Azee Bee Nahgha of Dine Nation Inc.,

Begay DH, Maryboy NC (2000) The whole universe is my cathedral: a contemporary Navajo spiritual synthesis. Med Anthropol Q 14(4):498–520

Begaye L (2017) Navajo Nation Department of behavioral health services recruitment and rentention initiative. Navajo Nation Department of Health

Brave Heart MY, DeBruyn LM (1998) The American Indian Holocaust: healing historical unresolved grief. Am Indian Alsk Native Mental Health Res 8(2):56–78

Cohen K (1998) Native American medicine. Altern Ther Health Med 4(6):45–57

Coyhis D, Simonelli R (2005) Rebuilding native American communities. Child Welfare 84(2):323–336

Donovan B (1997) Fake Healers Plague Navajo Nation. High Country News. 13 Oct 1997

Esposito M, Kahn-John M (2020) American Indian Traditional Medicine: navigation pathways for allopathic practice 2020

Goodkind JR, Hess JM, Gorman B, Parker DP (2012) "We're still in a struggle": Dine resilience, survival, historical trauma, and healing. Qual Health Res 22(8):1019–1036

Grandbois DM, Sanders GF (2009) The resilience of native American elders. Issues Ment Health Nurs 30(9):569–580

Hartmann WE, Gone JP (2014) American Indian historical trauma: community perspectives from two Great Plains medicine men. Am J Community Psychol 54(3–4):274–288

Heafner JC, Buchanan B (2016) Exploration of why Alaskans use complementary medicine: a focus group study. J Holist Nurs 34(2):200–211

Joe JR, Young RS, Moses J, Knoki-Wilson U, Dennison J (2016a) At the bedside: traditional Navajo practitioners in a patient-centered health care model. Am Indian Alsk Native Mental Health Res 23(2):28–49

Joe JR, Young RS, Moses J, Knoki-Wilson U, Dennison J (2016b) A collaborative case study: The Office of Native Medicine. Am Indian Alsk Native Mental Health Res 23(2):50–63

Kahn-John M (2010) Concept analysis of Dine Hozho: a Dine wellness philosophy. ANS Adv Nurs Sci 33(2):113–125

Kim C, Kwok YS (1998) Navajo use of native healers. Arch Intern Med 158(20):2245–2249

Moghaddam J, Momper S, Fong T (2015) Crystalizing the role of traditional healing in an urban native American Health Center. Community Ment Health J 51(3):305–314

Moorehead VD Jr, Gone JP, December D (2015) A gathering of native American healers: exploring the interface of indigenous tradition and professional practice. Am J Community Psychol 56(3–4):383–394

Moss M, Tibbetts L, Henly SJ, Dahlen BJ, Patchell B, Struthers R (2005) Strengthening American Indian nurse scientist training through tradition: partnering with elders. J Cult Divers 12(2):50–55

National Institutes of Health Tribal Health Research Office (NIH THRO) (2019) NIH. Traditional medicine summit: maintaining and protecting culture through healing: National Institutes of Health; 2019 [Website for the Traditional Medicine Summit sponsored by the National Institutes of Health Tribal Health Research Office, Indian Health Services, Centers for Disease Control and the Centers for Complementary and Alternative Medicine]. Available from: https://dpcpsi.nih.gov/thro/tms

Navajo CARES Act (2020) The original first responders should not be left out of Navajo CARES Act funding [press release]. 13 July 2020

Novins DK, Beals J, Moore LA, Spicer P, Manson SM (2004) Use of biomedical services and traditional healing options among American Indians: sociodemographic correlates, spirituality, and ethnic identity. Med Care 42(7):670–679

Redvers N, Blondin B (2020) Traditional Indigenous medicine in North America: A scoping review. PLoS ONE 15(8): e0237531. https://doi.org/10.1371/journal.pone.0237531

Southcentral Foundation (2020) Southcentral Foundation Traditional Healing Clinic (SCF). Available from: https://www.southcentralfoundation.com/services/traditional-healing/

Struthers R, Littlejohn S (1999) The essence of native American nursing. J Transcult Nurs 10(2):131–135

Struthers R, Eschiti VS, Patchell B (2004) Traditional indigenous healing: Part I. Complement Ther Nurs Midwifery 10(3):141–149

Struthers R, Lauderdale J, Nichols LA, Tom-Orme L, Strickland CJ (2005) Respecting tribal traditions in research and publications: voices of five native American nurse scholars. J Transcult Nurs 16(3):193–201

United States Department of Health and Human Health Services (2020a) Indian Health Services: IHS Profile Fact Sheet 2020. Available from: https://www.ihs.gov/newsroom/factsheets/ihsprofile/

United States Department of Health and Human Health Services (2020b) Complementary, alternative or integrative health: what's in a name? : National Center for Complementary and Alternative Health; 2020. Available from: https://www.nccih.nih.gov/health/complementary-alternative-or-integrative-health-whats-in-a-name

United States Department of Health and Human Health Services (2020c) About the Indian Health Services 2020. Available from: https://www.ihs.gov/aboutihs/overview/

United States Department of Health and Human Services (2020) Indian Health Services Disparities Fact Sheet 2020. Available from: https://www.ihs.gov/newsroom/factsheets/disparities/

Waldram JB (2013) Transformative and restorative processes: revisiting the question of efficacy of indigenous healing. Med Anthropol 32(3):191–207

Whitbeck LB, Adams GW, Hoyt DR, Chen X (2004) Conceptualizing and measuring historical trauma among American Indian people. Am J Community Psychol 33(3–4):119–130

World Health Organization (2013) WHO Traditional Medicine Strategy: 2014–2023. Available from: https://www.who.int/traditional-complementary-integrative-medicine/publications/trm_strategy14_23/en/areas/traditional/definitions/en/)

World Health Organization (2019) WHO global report on traditional and complementary medicine 2019. Available from: https://apps.who.int/iris/handle/10665/312342

Role of Nature Therapy and Mindfulness for Resilience Among Rural Healthcare Providers

16

Christina Harlow

> *In the presence of nature, a wild delight runs through the man, in spite of real sorrows. Nature says, -- he is my creature, and maugre all his impertinent griefs, he shall be glad with me.*
>
> —Ralph Waldo Emerson

16.1 Introduction

As healthcare providers of all disciplines, we are taught to educate our patients to care for themselves through lifestyle changes such as diet, exercise, and sleep. Our approach to healing is often focused on symptom management. As integrative healthcare providers, we accept a more global approach to the human experience and consider their wellbeing in addition to lifestyle, and the focus shifts away from symptoms and onto patient-centered outcomes. As healthcare providers in rural settings, our patients tend to be sicker, poorer, and less likely to be able to achieve wellness for a variety of reasons. We ourselves may be sicker, more burned out, with many fewer resources. This not only impacts our own health, but has significant implications for the outcomes of our patients. This chapter discusses the evidence behind these concepts and offers some recommendations for both personal wellbeing and patient wellbeing.

C. Harlow (✉)
University of Vermont, Burlington, VT, USA
e-mail: charlow@giffordhealthcare.org

© Springer Nature Switzerland AG 2021
A. Vermeesch (ed.), *Integrative Health Nursing Interventions for Vulnerable Populations*, https://doi.org/10.1007/978-3-030-60043-3_16

16.2   Philosophical Underpinnings

One of the foundational principles of integrative nursing is, "Nature has healing and restorative properties that contribute to health and wellbeing." This aligns closely with the first principle of integrative nursing, which is "Human beings are whole systems, inseparable from their environments" (Kreitzer and Koithan 2014). The second integrative nursing principle is, "Human beings have the innate capacity for health and wellbeing." These principles are the philosophical underpinning of this chapter because while innately we understand nature is good for us, we learn how the natural environment is interwoven with our very existence, and therefore has a profound impact on our state of wellbeing. In addition, we all have the capacity to achieve health and wellbeing ourselves, and we can inspire these in our patients by building a strong relationship and giving them tools to help them both define and become what wellbeing means to them. So, what exactly is "wellbeing"? For the purpose of this book chapter, wellbeing is highly individualized, where the person achieves where they want to be in regard to physical, emotional, mental, environmental, and spiritual health. What is wellbeing for you may not be the same for your patients. The role of the integrative nurse, when considering these principles, is to apply not only "routine" nursing interventions, but to give attention to a patient's clarity and purpose, overall wellbeing, happiness, and energy (Kreitzer and Koithan 2019). Ultimately, when the integrative provider considers the person in front of them as complex with a dynamic expression of symptoms, beliefs, experiences, and personal ideas of wellbeing; both the practitioner and the patient will reap tremendous benefit. It is equally important that we consider our own wellbeing, as while the field of medicine brings satisfaction, it also brings burnout.

16.3   Background and Definitions

There is no general consensus on the definition of "rurality"; however, population density and distance from urban centers are commonly factors designating a rural area (Schlairet 2017). For this chapter, we consider rurality in the context of small healthcare facilities, likely designated as "critical access," caring for a population that is spread over a large land area and far from an urban center. In consideration of vulnerable populations, it is known that living rurally is a risk factor for health disparities such as socio-economic disparities and racial disparities such as being a migrant farm worker. There is substantial research into the state of rurality contributing to health disparities, but less is known about how the healthcare providers that balance caring for vulnerable populations manage their own health, particularly their increased risk of burnout.

Before COVID-19 impacted how we approach healthcare, studies reported that over 50% of American physicians on the "frontline" (emergency medicine, family medicine, internal medicine) were experiencing significant levels of burnout. These statistics are congruent with burnout levels in non-physician providers (nurse practitioners, physician assistants) and nurses as well. This is significant because not only is the provider's own physical and mental health dramatically affected, it has serious implications for patient safety and satisfaction (Waddimba et al. 2015). It is also significant because while data is not yet available, it is highly likely that levels of burnout in healthcare workers are significantly higher during and following the pandemic. When a provider is practicing in a rural area, the risk of burnout is increased substantially because of constraints in resources, salaries, and isolation (social, organizational, and/or geographic). Additionally, patients tend to be sicker and have fewer resources themselves which leads to distressing interactions (Stevenson et al. 2011). Many urban and large hospital systems are addressing burnout with wellness programs that include support groups, access to gyms, and other initiatives. Rural and remote practice areas often do not have the resources to provide substantial support to their personnel, and it is not common for organizations with less than 1000 employees to provide a comprehensive wellness program (Baicker et al. 2010).

Nature therapy is a term loosely used to define several different approaches to establishing a therapeutic environment while in nature (Berger 2009). Several methods and approaches have been researched extensively. For this book chapter, we primarily focus on a specific form of nature therapy called forest bathing, or Shinrin-Yoku. Forest bathing (shinrin-yoku) was developed in Japan in 1982 by the Ministry of Agriculture, and has been studied primarily in Japan but is becoming increasingly practiced and researched all over the world (Wen et al. 2019). Forest bathing approaches the therapeutic environment through the five senses (vision, hearing, taste, smell, and touch) as a person is immersed in nature, preferably with trees. Much of the current evidence is focused on how forest bathing affects both physical and mental health, specifically immunity, stress, and mood conditions such as depression and anxiety (Hansen et al. 2017). There is substantial evidence that forest bathing increases natural killer cells hence boosting immunity, decreases cortisol levels and blood pressure, and decreases both anxiety and depression.

Mindfulness in the context of this chapter is defined as, "purposeful and nonjudgmental attentiveness to one's own experience, thoughts, and feelings" (Beach et al. 2013). As symptoms of burnout have been found to substantially affect patient outcomes negatively, practicing mindfulness has the exact opposite effect, and patient outcomes improve. There is a gap in evidence evaluating mindfulness training in rural healthcare providers although a few recent studies have reported improvements in self-compassion and resilience following mindfulness training. One study evaluated an online mindfulness approach, which may be a viable method for rural healthcare providers (Moore et al. 2020).

Resilience is a fluid trait that is defined as the ability to adapt in a positive manner when faced with adversity (Robertson et al. 2016). Stephens (2013) defines resilience as an individual process of development that occurs through the use of personal protective factors to successfully navigate perceived stress and adversities. This resilience leads to improved coping and adaptive abilities as well as increased wellbeing (Stephens 2013). Resilience is a key component of provider satisfaction in both rural and urban areas and has an inverse relationship with burnout as does mindfulness.

16.4 Current Evidence and Recommendations

Forest bathing is considered a vital piece of healthy living in parts of Asia, and the growing body of evidence is finding significant, replicable health benefits, though more research is needed—particularly outside of Asia—to evaluate clinically significant outcomes (Hansen et al. 2017). Physiological elements that have been found to benefit from forest bathing include cardiopulmonary improvements, increases in natural killer cells both short and extended term after nature immersion, and mental health benefits, specifically anxiety and stress reduction (Hansen et al. 2017). There is no current consensus on prescribing forest bathing in the clinical setting, but experts recommend 2 h of nature immersion for best results, but sessions as short as 20 min have been found to have positive benefits (Li 2018). Forest bathing, as previously mentioned, is a mindfulness practice. It is imperative that one walks slowly, quietly, pausing to observe and absorb the natural environment with all senses (Li 2018). There are now several studies that have evaluated stress responses after forest bathing by measuring salivary cortisol levels and biophysical markers such as heart rate and blood pressure (Li 2018). Consistently and routinely, forest bathing is found to decrease stress levels (Hansen et al. 2017). Perhaps the most provocative benefit from forest bathing is the evidence for improving immune function, particularly by the increase of natural killer (NK) cells (Miyazaki 2018). This increase in NK cells is improved for several days, implying lasting benefit from forest bathing (Li 2010). These physiological benefits of forest bathing are important and can contribute to overall wellbeing of our patients and ourselves (see Fig. 16.1). Figure 16.1 is a short guide to forest bathing for preparation and use for providers and lay individuals. Perhaps even more important is the mental and emotional benefits of forest bathing, when considering avoiding healthcare provider burnout. Forest bathing is meditative and the benefits of mindfulness are reaped.

16.5 Conclusion

In conclusion, rural healthcare providers are at an increased risk of burnout when compared to their urban colleagues, and a growing body of evidence finds that this is minimized somewhat by having innate resilience traits. Furthermore, training providers in mindfulness techniques is promising to also lessen the burden of burnout. Spending time in nature, particularly in a state of mindfulness, has many physical and mental health benefits and this, dear readers, is what I believe is the golden ticket. John Muir famously said, "into the woods I go, to lose my mind and find my soul." As a rural healthcare provider myself, nothing rings more true than this sentiment during the COVID-19 pandemic. If contextually, we embrace the integrative nursing principles in our approach to not only ourselves but our patients, we understand not only that each person is complex, but also has an innate ability to heal oneself, and most certainly benefits from being in nature.

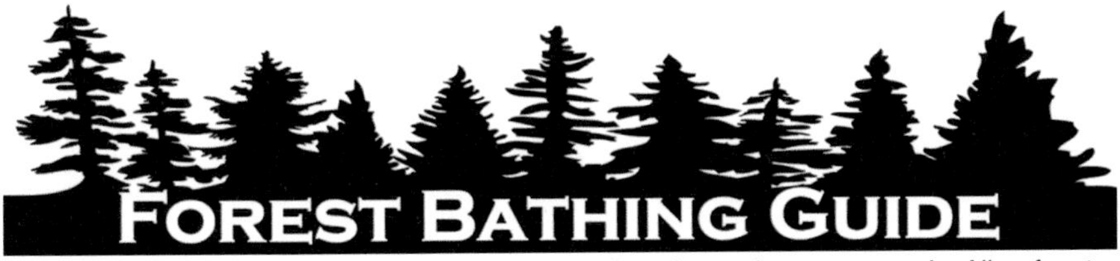

Preparation: Leave behind all distractions, including electronics, pets, people. Allow for at least 20 minutes and up to 2 hours for experience. Leave all expectations at home. Find a tree, or many trees, and enter with open heart and mind.

Sensory Experience	Tools/Recommendations
Visual	Look for light through the trees, different colors, animals, textures. What do you see? Reflect.
Auditory	Listen for silence. Listen for wind, animals, your breath. What else do you hear? Reflect.
Olfactory	Pick up a flower, pine needle, or other natural object. Does it have a scent? What do you smell in the air? Reflect.
Tactile	Remove your shoes if possible. How does the ground feel? Touch tree bark, leaves, twigs, flowers. How are their textures different? What subtleties do you find? Reflect.
Taste	Bring warm tea, preferably made of local herbs or plants. If not available herbal tea works as well. How does it taste? What plant is it made from? Reflect.

Fig. 16.1 Forest bathing guide (© Harlow, 2020). (Developed for the purpose of this book by Christina Harlow DNP, FNP-BC)

References

Baicker K, Cutler D, Song Z (2010) Workplace wellness programs can generate savings. Health Aff 29:304–311

Bas-Sarmiento P, Fernández-Gutiérrez M, Baena-Baños M, Romero-Sánchez JM (2017) Efficacy of empathy training in nursing students: a quasi-experimental study. Nurse Educ Today 59:59–65

Beach MC, Roter D, Korthuis PT et al (2013) A multicenter study of physician mindfulness and health care quality. Ann Fam Med 11:421–428

Berger R (2009) Nature therapy: thoughts about the limitations of practice. J Humanist Psychol 50:65–76

Clifford MA (2018) Your guide to forest bathing: experience the healing power of nature. Conari Press, Newburyport

Djernis L, Poulsen S, Dahlgaard O'T (2019) A systematic review and meta-analysis of nature-based mindfulness: effects of moving mindfulness training into an outdoor natural setting. Int J Environ Res Public Health 16:3202

Hansen MM, Jones R, Tocchini K (2017) Shinrin-Yoku (Forest bathing) and nature therapy: a state-of-the-art review. Int J Environ Res Public Health 14:851

Kreitzer M, Koithan M (2014) Integrative Nursing. Oxford University Press

Li Q (2010) Effect of forest bathing trips on human immune function. Environmental Health and Preventive Medicine 15:9–17

Li Q (2018) Forest bathing: how trees can help you find health and happiness. Viking

Li Y, Cao F, Cao D, Liu J (2014) Nursing students' post-traumatic growth, emotional intelligence and psychological resilience. J Psychiatr Ment Health Nurs 22:326–332

Madewell AN, Ponce-Garcia E (2016) Assessing resilience in emerging adulthood: the Resilience Scale (RS), Connor–Davidson Resilience Scale (CD-RISC), and Scale of Protective Factors (SPF). Personal Individ Differ 97:249–255

Miyazaki Y (2018) Shinrin Yoku: the Japanese art of forest bathing. Storey Publishing, LLC, North Adams, MA

Moore SJ, Barbour R, Ngo H, Sinclair C, Chambers R, Auret K, Hassed C, Playford D (2020) Determining the feasibility and effectiveness of brief online mindfulness training for rural medical students: a pilot study. BMC Med Educ 20:104. https://doi.org/10.21203/rs.2.13728/v1

Pines EW, Rauschhuber ML, Norgan GH, Cook JD, Canchola L, Richardson C, Jones ME (2012) Stress resiliency, psychological empowerment and conflict management styles among baccalaureate nursing students. J Adv Nurs 68:1482–1493

Rahim S (2013) Clinical application of Nightingale's environmental theory. i-manager's J Nurs 3:43–46

Robertson HD, Elliott AM, Burton C, Iversen L, Murchie P, Porteous T, Matheson C (2016) Resilience of primary healthcare professionals: a systematic review. Br J Gen Pract 66(647):e423–e433. https://doi.org/10.3399/bjgp16x685261

Schlairet MC (2017) Complexity compression in rural nursing. Online J Rural Nurs Health Care 17:2–33

Stephens TM (2013) Nursing student resilience: a concept clarification. Nurs Forum 48:125–133

Stevenson AD, Phillips CB, Anderson KJ (2011) Resilience among doctors who work in challenging areas: a qualitative study. Br J Gen Pract 61(588):e404–e410. https://doi.org/10.3399/bjgp11x583182

Waddimba AC, Scribani M, Nieves MA, Krupa N, May JJ, Jenkins P (2015) Validation of single-item screening measures for provider burnout in a rural health care network. Eval Health Prof 39:215–225

Ward J, Cody J, Schaal M, Hojat M (2012) The empathy enigma: an empirical study of decline in empathy among undergraduate nursing students. J Prof Nurs 28:34–40

Wen Y, Yan Q, Pan Y, Gu X, Liu Y (2019) Medical empirical research on forest bathing (Shinrin-yoku): a systematic review. Environ Health Prev Med 24(1):70. https://doi.org/10.1186/s12199-019-0822-8

Veteran Health Care and Special Considerations

17

Fernando Carrillo and Patricia Cox

17.1 Introduction

There are over 20 million veterans in the United States of which 18 million are male and approximately two million are female (U.S. Department of Veterans Affairs 2020a). Military personnel and military veterans have unique health concerns as a result of injuries, combat, multiple deployments, and environmental exposures. Not all veterans obtain health care from the U.S. Department of Veterans Affairs (VA). Only those who received either a general or honorable discharge may qualify for health care benefits. In fiscal year 2017, about 49% of all veterans used at least one VA benefit which is an 11% increase in utilization since 2008 (U.S. Department of Veterans Affairs 2020b).

The Centers for Disease Control and Prevention (2012) reported veterans were more likely than nonveterans to vocalize they had fair or poor health. This was particularly true in veterans who were younger (45–54 years of age) who identified themselves as having two or more chronic conditions versus older nonveterans aged 45–64 who had one or none of these chronic conditions. Veterans, when compared to nonveterans, also reported more psychological distress and experiencing work limitations more often.

In 2017, the median age of male veterans in the United States was 65, while the median age of male nonveterans was 42. Like their male counterparts, female veterans are also older with a median age of 51 compared to nonveteran females with a median age of 47 (U.S. Department of Veterans Affairs 2019). The need to care for veterans will continue to grow over time as this population advances in age and experiences a higher burden for both acute and chronic illnesses across the continuum of hospitals, outpatient clinics, and long-term care. Furthermore, comparisons

F. Carrillo
Primary Care Division, Portland VA Medical Center, Vancouver, WA, USA
e-mail: Luis.Carrillo3@va.gov

P. Cox (✉)
School of Nursing, University of Portland, Portland, OR, USA
e-mail: coxp@up.edu

© Springer Nature Switzerland AG 2021
A. Vermeesch (ed.), *Integrative Health Nursing Interventions for Vulnerable Populations*, https://doi.org/10.1007/978-3-030-60043-3_17

of health differences between veterans and nonveterans over the age of 65 and older suggest that the effects of military service on health may appear in veterans later in life (Wilmoth et al. 2010).

With recent medical and technological advances, more veterans have survived injuries from wars that in earlier conflicts would have killed them (Morin 2011). For example, the signature wound caused by improvised explosive devices (IED) in the post-September 11 wars resulted in polytraumatic injuries, including multiple limb loss, burns, spinal cord injury, traumatic brain injury (TBI), facial trauma, and blindness (Belmont et al. 2012; Ramasamy et al. 2011). Some of these injuries often are deadly, and if someone survives them, treatment is often costly and requires long-term rehabilitation (Gray et al. 2017).

The average American can expect to live to age 78.6 with women outliving men by comparison 81.1 years versus 76.1 years, respectively (Centers for Disease Control and Prevention 2019). If the mean average age of service members who suffered polytraumatic injuries is 26 (Belmont et al. 2012), and because of their youth and their likelihood of having a similar life expectancy to other Americans, then it is feasible they may live another 50 years with one or more chronic conditions. As they grow older, veterans from recent wars will face secondary and tertiary consequences. An amputee, for instance, may experience decreased mobility, which can result in weight gain, leading to diabetes, and culminating in cardiovascular disease. Another example are veterans who experience Post-Traumatic Stress Disorder (PTSD); they may also gain weight, use tobacco, suffer depression, or develop substance abuse disorders. All of which will diminish longevity and quality of life. Nurses involved in the care of veterans, whether through the VA or in the community, can use resources outlined in this chapter to guide their interventions.

17.2 Why Is It Important?

Men and women will continue to serve in the U.S. Armed Forces and become veterans who will need care as they age and as a result of their military service. The American Nurses Association, American Association of Nurse Practitioners, American Association of Colleges of Nursing, and the Nation League for Nursing, in conjunction with the Department of Veterans Affairs support the practice of nurses asking all patients whether they are veterans (The White House 2012). Moreover, nursing philosophy places the patient at the center of their own care with nurses striving to collaborate with the patient to achieve the best outcomes. Therefore, it is paramount that nurses understand who a veteran is, recognize the health issues facing veterans, and identify what services are available to them.

17.3 Who Is a Veteran?

Title 38 of the Code of Federal Regulations defines who is a veteran. Under this code, a veteran is a person who served in the active military, naval, or air service and who was discharged or released under conditions other than dishonorable.

Consequently, individuals who completed service in any branch of the United States Armed Forces (Army, Air Force, Navy, Marine Corp, and Coast Guard, including their Reserve components) are veterans unless they received a dishonorable discharge (Electronic Code of Federal Regulations 2020). For more information on the eligibility and benefits, please contact your local VA (see Appendix).

17.4 What Is Whole Health?

In 2011, the VA transformed and reoriented their disease-focused health system to one that focuses on the well-being of the veteran. This redesign is veteran driven. Its goal is for veterans to move beyond seeing themselves as patients and to see themselves as people defining their own health goals, whether it is for them to interpret health as being able to bend over to tie their own shoes, or perhaps reaching the soaring goal of running a marathon, or anything in between (Gaudet and Kligler 2019). The concept of Whole Health focuses on what matters most to the veteran and not what matters most to his or her health care providers. Whole Health recognizes the importance of healthy diet, physical activity, sleep, relationships, surroundings, and all the other areas of life that contribute to someone's health and well-being (University of Wisconsin-Madison 2020).

The keystone of Whole Health is to blend conventional medicine together with such integrative health modalities as self-care, mindfulness, yoga, Tai Chi, and acupuncture. The Circle of Health (see Fig. 17.1) guides veterans as they reflect on their own health and well-being while participating in discussions with members of their own care teams, rather than being passive recipients of care directed by clinicians (University of Wisconsin-Madison 2020).

17.5 Vignette

The following vignette is a conversation shared between a veteran and you, the nurse of his care team. Whole Health concepts will be integrated throughout the following example to illustrate the use of integrative modalities:

Mark is a 48-year-old who served in the U.S. Army soon after 9/11. He received an honorable discharge after serving his country for 6 years. He works as a phlebotomist and lives with his wife and daughter. During a clinic visit, he tells you that he feels anxious, angry, and hypervigilant. He also complains of daily headaches. These symptoms affect his work performance, as well as his relationship with his wife and daughter. He confides in you that he was sexually assaulted during his military service. He has never shared this information with anyone before. Not even his wife. Mark is likely experiencing symptoms of post-traumatic stress disorder and military sexual trauma.

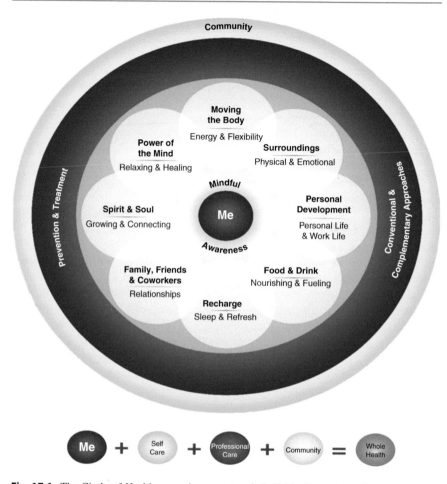

Fig. 17.1 The Circle of Health recognizes a veteran's individuality, putting the veteran at the center. The veteran is empowered by mindfulness and self-care. The care team and the community support and embrace the veteran by using both conventional and complementary modalities. When veterans use the Circle of Health, they can identify what matters most to them, so they can talk to their care team to move closer to reach set health goals. Accessed 23 July 2020 https://wholehealth. wisc.edu/

17.6 Post-Traumatic Stress Disorder

Post-traumatic stress disorder is a common, complex, and serious disorder affecting veterans from every conflict. For instance, 11% of veterans who served in either Operations Iraqi Freedom or Enduring Freedom, 12% of veterans who in Desert Storm, and 15% of veterans who served in Vietnam suffer from PTSD (U.S. Department of Veterans Affairs 2020c). PTSD is a somatic, a cognitive, a behavioral, and an affective disorder. Veterans with PTSD, like Mark in our vignette, experience hypervigilance, nightmares, intrusive thoughts, flashbacks of past traumatic events, and sleep disorders. These symptoms lead to social, occupational, and interpersonal problems. Although trauma can be a life-changing event, veterans are resilient, and many will recover without professional help. Others may function well in their life, but they continue to experience some level of difficulties or have strong reactions in certain situations. The diagnosis of PTSD is difficult to confirm because the presentation of symptoms can vary. A complicating factor is that traumatic events are associated with a range of other psychopathology, including depression and anxiety disorders. Examples of traumatic events common in veterans include combat, sexual assault (similar to Mark), physical injury or medical illness, and mass conflict and displacement (U.S. Department of Veterans Affairs 2020d).

Treatment for PTSD ideally should start soon after diagnosis and focuses on recovery with attention to the veterans' needs and preferences to help them fulfill their personal goals and live meaningful lives. For most veterans, treatment is trauma-focused psychotherapy, cognitive behavioral therapy, or a combination of both. Trauma-focused therapy is an approach to understand how the traumatic experience impacts mental, behavioral, emotional, physical, and spiritual well-being. The goal of trauma-focused therapy is to offer skills and strategies to assist veterans in better understanding, coping with, processing emotions and memories tied to traumatic experiences, thus enabling veterans to create a healthier and more adaptive meaning of the experience that took place in their life. Exposure therapy is used together with relaxation exercises and guided imagery. This helps veterans learn how to bring about a relaxed state at-will, while gradually exposing them to what they fear and helps them cope. Along with psychotherapy, the use of antidepressants may improve signs and symptoms of PTSD. Mark, like other veterans, would benefit from these modalities (U.S. Department of Veterans Affairs 2020e). See Appendix for more information resources, and who to contact in case of a mental health crisis.

Another intervention to enhance self-care and manage PTSD symptoms is the use of mobile apps (Owen et al. 2018). Mark could benefit from using either the PTSD Coach and the Mindfulness Coach apps or both. His wife may also benefit from the PTSD Family Coach, which is designed for loved ones of those with PTSD. The VA makes these apps available free of charge to both veterans and the general public. These tools provide veterans and their loved ones with quick, easy-to-use tools and direct links to additional support (U.S. Department of Veterans Affairs 2020f). With the wide use of smartphones, Mark can download the app to his mobile device, which provides him with easy access and privacy as he can carry his smartphone with him anywhere he goes.

17.7   Military Sexual Trauma

One in four women and 1 in 100 men report Military Sexual Trauma (MST). These numbers only reflect the rates of MST in veterans who choose to seek health care in the VA; therefore, the true rate of sexual assault or harassment among all veterans who have served is unknown (VA Health Care 2015).

In the vignette, Mark confides for the first time that he experienced military sexual trauma. The VA defines MST as acts of sexual assault or sexual harassment experienced by veterans during their military service. The definition originates from Title 38 U.S. Code 1720D, which describes MST as a psychological trauma from battery, physical assault, or harassment of a sexual nature. MST includes any sexual activity where service members are involved against their will, cannot consent to engaging in sexual activities, or are forced into sexual activities (VA Health Care 2015). Other types of MST include:

- Unwanted sexual touching or grabbing.
- Offensive remarks about a person's body.
- Unwelcomed sexual advances.

It is important to keep in mind that not all veterans who experienced MST need or are interested in treatment. MST is neither a diagnosis nor a mental health condition. To help veterans feel more at ease and talk frankly about their own experiences with MST, veterans can ask to meet with a clinician of a specific gender, if it would make them feel more comfortable.

Mark experienced MST and has unique needs, so treatment goals will focus on helping him meet his aspirations and improve the severity of his symptoms. The severity and duration of Mark's difficulties with MST will vary based on his prior history of trauma and whether it happened once or repeatedly. Although the reactions between men and women who have MST are similar in some ways, survivors of both genders struggle with different issues. Factors such as race and ethnicity, religion, sexual orientation, and other cultural variables can affect the impact of MST (VA Health Care 2015). See Table 17.1 for other symptoms and behaviors resulting from MST that both female and male survivors may experience.

The VA is committed to helping veterans receive the care they need to recover from MST. Every VA across the nation has a designated MST Coordinator who serves as a contact, and helps veterans find and access VA services, state and federal benefits, and community resources. For more information, veterans can speak with their VA health care provider, get in touch with their local Vet Center, or contact the MST Coordinator at their nearest VA (see Appendix).

17.8   Chronic Pain

According to National Center for Complementary and Integrative Health, veterans experienced higher pain severity than nonveterans in a previous three-month period. These results show the disparity between severe pain related to painful health conditions in veterans and nonveterans (see Fig. 17.2). If we consider gender in the experience of severe pain (see Fig. 17.3), male veterans were more

Table 17.1 Other symptoms and behaviors, which result from military sexual trauma that both female and male survivors may experience

Feeling depressed	Intense, sudden emotional reaction to situations	Feeling angry or irritable all the time	Feeling emotionally flat
Difficulty experiencing emotions like love or happiness	Trouble falling or staying asleep or disturbing nightmares	Trouble staying focused	Finding their mild wandering
Having difficulties remembering things	Drinking alcohol to excess or using drugs daily	Getting intoxicated or high to cope with memories or emotional reactions	Drinking to fall asleep
Feeling on edge all the time	Difficulty feeling safe	Going out of their way to avoid reminders of their experiences	Feeling isolated or disconnected from others
Staying in abusive relationships	Having trouble with employers or authority figures	Having difficulty with trusting others	Experiencing sexual difficulties
Having chronic pain	Gaining weight	Eating problems	Having gastrointestinal problems

likely to report any pain when compared to male nonveterans and to have higher rates of severe pain. Female veterans were also more likely to report any pain than female nonveterans; however, there was no difference in the proportion between the two groups of female participants who reported severe pain (National Institutes of Health 2020).

Pain is a common reason to seek medical care. It is one of the top reasons why veterans turn to integrative health approaches. To clarify, we need to recognize the differences between acute and chronic pain because understanding the differences helps shift how pain is managed and how physical functioning is preserved. Acute pain is a normal sensation to injury, it is time limited, and it signals the need to take care of the injured site; for example, an acute ankle sprain might be managed by immobilization for a short time. Chronic pain, in contrast, is much different because chronic pain persists despite self-care, and it seldom improves with the use of chronic opioids. One of the goals of chronic pain management is preserving or improving physical functioning. Common chronic pain complaints include headache, low back, arthritis, neurogenic, and psychogenic pain. Some of these conditions can be treated successfully by physical therapy, massage, stretching exercises, occupational therapy, relaxation techniques such as deep breathing or meditation, biofeedback, and transcutaneous electrical nerve stimulation. For some veterans, chronic pain exists despite the absence of injury or evidence of body damage; for example, Mark complains of daily headaches, which can be attributed to his PTSD and exacerbated by his MST. In one study, the 12-month PTSD prevalence rate in

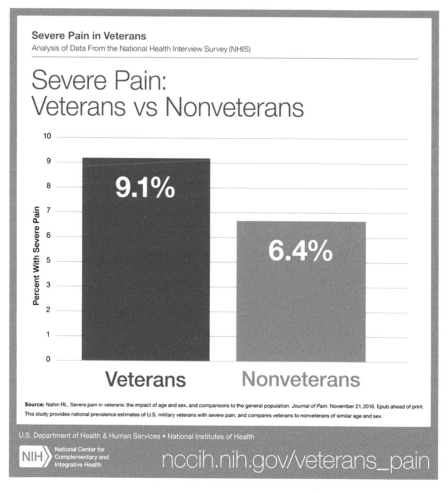

Fig. 17.2 Veterans were more likely to report having any pain in the prior 3 months than nonveterans. Accessed 24 July 2020 from https://www.nccih.nih.gov/health/pain/veterans

study participants who suffered headaches was 14.3%, while the lifetime PTSD prevalence rate was 21.5%. On the other hand, study participants without headaches had a PTSD prevalence rate of 2.1% (12-month) and 4.5% (lifetime). Of note, the study showed that PTSD symptoms triggered headaches in almost 70% of those study participants who reported headaches and PTSD. As far as treatment options for Mark, behavioral treatment alone has been shown to positively influence chronic pain and disability in people with PTSD. Therefore, the use of cognitive behavioral therapy, alone or in combination with pharmacological therapy, could be considered (American Headache Society n.d.).

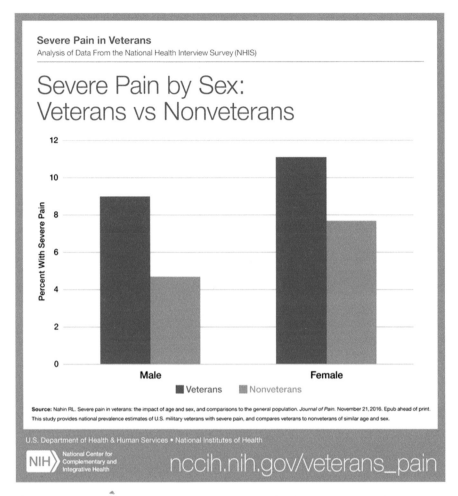

Fig. 17.3 Male veterans were more likely to report any pain when compared to male nonveterans and to have higher rates of severe pain. Female veterans were also more likely to report any pain than female nonveterans; however, there was no difference in the proportion between the two groups of female participants who reported severe pain. Accessed 24 July 2020, from https://www. nccih.nih.gov/health/pain/veterans

17.9   Conclusion

Mark presents with chronic headaches, PTSD, and MST. Traditionally, nurses who practice within a disease-driven model consider the absence of disease as success in providing care; however, this is not always an attainable goal. More important, nursing philosophy places the person at the center of their own care with nurses striving to collaborate with the individual to achieve the best outcome. Ultimately, when nurses incorporate the concept of Whole Health into their practice, veterans such as

Mark can use their own self-care strategies to promote their own health and strengthen their own innate healing ability. Thus, Mark—and other veterans like him—can strive to reach their potential whatever that may be.

Appendix

U.S. Department of Veterans Affairs
Find VA Locations
Call: (844) 698–2311
Website: http://www.va.gov
Vet Centers
Vet Centers are community-based counseling centers that provide a wide range of social and psychological services, including professional readjustment counseling.
Call: (877) WAR-VETS (927-8387)
Website: https://www.vetcenter.va.gov
Veterans Crisis Line (24/7)
The Veterans Crisis Line is a free, confidential resource available to anyone. Qualified responders at the Veterans Crisis Line are trained and experienced in helping veterans of all ages and circumstances.
Call: (800) 273-8255, Press 1
Text: 838255
For hearing impaired, call TTY (800) 799-4889
Website/Chat Online: https://www.veteranscrisisline.net
Military Sexual Trauma
Coping suggestions and resources for connecting with care for military sexual trauma survivors and others feeling pain and distress due to recent events related to military sexual trauma.
Website: https://www.mentalhealth.va.gov/msthome/resources.asp
To Find Local Military Sexual Trauma Coordinator
Website: https://www.benefits.va.gov/benefits/mstcoordinators.asp
Make the Connection
This is an online resource designed to connect veterans, their family members, friends, and other supporters with information, resources, and solutions to issues affecting their lives.
Website: https://maketheconnection.net

References

American Headache Society (n.d.) Post-traumatic stress disorder (PTSD) & migraine. https://americanheadachesociety.org/news/post-traumatic-stress-disorder-ptsd-migraine/. Accessed 24 July 2020

Belmont, P.J., McCriskin, B.J., Sieg, R.N., Burks, R. & Schoenfeld, A.J. (2012). Combat wounds in Iraq and Afghanistan from 2005 to 2009. J Trauma Acute Care Surg 73(1):3–12. https://journals.lww.com/jtrauma/Abstract/2012/07000/Combat_wounds_in_Iraq_and_Afghanistan_from_2005_to.2.aspx. Accessed 25 July 2020

Centers for Disease Control and Prevention (2012) The health of male veterans and nonveterans aged 25–64: United States, 2007–2010. National Center for Health Statistics Data Brief, No. 101, August 2012. https://www.cdc.gov/nchs/products/databriefs/db101.htm. Accessed 23 July 2020

Centers for Disease Control and Prevention (2019) National Center for Health Statistics. Health, United States, 2018 data finder. https://www.cdc.gov/nchs/data/hus/2018/004.pdf. Accessed 23 July 2020

Electronic Code of Federal Regulations (2020) Title 38: pensions, bonuses, and veterans' relief, part 3 adjudication: general, Section 3.1. https://www.ecfr.gov/cgi-bin/text-idx?SID=2c2 7136e25a56c5230cdd3f952acd6dc&node=pt38.1.3&rgn=div5#se38.1.3_11. Accessed 23 July 2020

Gaudet T, Kligler B (2019) Whole health in the whole system of the veterans administration: how will we know we have reached this future state? J Altern Complement Med 25:S7–S11. https://www.liebertpub.com/doi/10.1089/acm.2018.29061.gau. Accessed 23 July 2020

Gray M, Chung J, Aguila F, Williams TG, Teraoka JK, Harris OA (2017) Long-term functional outcomes in military service members and veterans after traumatic brain injury/polytrauma inpatient rehabilitation. Arch Phys Med Rehabil 99(2):S33–S39. https://www.archives-pmr.org/article/S0003-9993(17)31023-7/fulltext#back-bib2. Accessed 25 July 2020

Morin R (2011) For many injured veterans, a lifetime of consequences. Pew Research Center. https://www.pewsocialtrends.org/2011/11/08/section-2-injured-post-911-veterans/. Accessed 25 July 2020

National Institute of Health (2020) National Center for Complementary and Integrative Health. Veterans endure higher pain severity than nonveterans. https://www.nccih.nih.gov/news/press-releases/veterans-endure-higher-pain-severity-than-nonveterans. Accessed 23 July 2020

Owen JE, Kuhn E, Jaworski BK, McGee-Vincent P, Juhasz K, Hoffman JE, Rosen C (2018) VA mobile apps for PTSD and related problems: public health resources for veterans and those who care for them. mHealth 4:28. https://doi.org/10.21037/mhealth.2018.05.07

Ramasamy A, Masouros SD, Newell N, Hill AM, Proud WG, Brown KA, Bull AM, Clasper JC (2011) In-vehicle extremity injuries from improvised explosive devices: current and future foci. Philos Trans R Soc Lond B Biol Sci 366(1562):160–170. https://doi.org/10.1098/rstb.2010.0219

The White House (2012) Office of the First Lady, America's nurses join forces with First Lady and Dr. Biden to support veterans and military families, 11 April 2012. Accessed from https://obamawhitehouse.archives.gov/the-press-office/2012/04/11/americas-nurses-join-forces-first-lady-and-dr-biden-support-veterans-and

U.S. Department of Veterans Affairs (2019) National Center for Veterans Analysis and Statistics: profile of veterans 2017. https://www.va.gov/vetdata/docs/SpecialReports/Profile_of_Veterans_2017.pdf. Accessed 23 July 2020

U.S. Department of Veterans Affairs (2020a) National Center for Veterans Analysis and Statistics: population tables: the nation age/gender. https://www.va.gov/vetdata/Veteran_Population.asp. Accessed 23 July 2020

U.S. Department of Veterans Affairs (2020b) National Center for Veterans Analysis and Statistics: VA utilization profile 2017. https://www.va.gov/vetdata/docs/Quickfacts/VA_Utilization_Profile_2017.pdf. Accessed 23 July 2020

U.S. Department of Veterans Affairs (2020c) National Center for PTSD. How common is PTSD in Veterans? https://www.ptsd.va.gov/understand/common/common_veterans.asp. Accessed 23 July 2020

U.S. Department of Veterans Affairs (2020d). National Center for PTSD. PTSD basics. https://www.ptsd.va.gov/understand/what/ptsd_basics.asp. Accessed 23 July 2020

U.S. Department of Veterans Affairs (2020e). National Center for PTSD. PTSD treatment basics. https://www.ptsd.va.gov/understand_tx/tx_basics.asp. Accessed 23 July 2020

U.S. Department of Veterans Affairs (2020f). National Center for PTSD. PTSD coach. https://www.ptsd.va.gov/appvid/mobile/ptsdcoach_app.asp. Accessed 23 July 2020

University of Wisconsin-Madison (2020) Whole health library: Advancing skills in the delivery of personalized, proactive, and patient-driven care. https://wholehealth.wisc.edu/. Accessed 23 July 2020

VA Health Care (2015) Military sexual trauma. https://www.mentalhealth.va.gov/docs/mst_general_factsheet.pdf. Accessed 23 July 2020

Wilmoth, J. M., London, A.S., & Parker, W. M. (2010). Military service and men's health trajectories in later life. J Gerontol B Psychol Sci Soc Sci, 65(6), 744–755. https://doi.org/10.1093/geronb/gbq072. Accessed 23 July 2020

Conclusion

Amber Vermeesch

With grit and grace, we move forward with our precious work to provide accessible tools for educators, practitioners, clinicians, researchers, and students to optimize the health of vulnerable populations globally. This work is by no means complete, yet we hope that it is useful in framing and tailoring appropriate interventions to better serve those among us who are vulnerable. Healthcare is a human right and together we strive for optimal, integrative wellness. After all, we are the healers, the action takers, the educators, and the pathfinders.

A. Vermeesch
School of Nursing, University of Portland, Portland, OR, USA

© Springer Nature Switzerland AG 2021
A. Vermeesch (ed.), *Integrative Health Nursing Interventions for Vulnerable Populations*, https://doi.org/10.1007/978-3-030-60043-3